FASTING FOR WOMEN

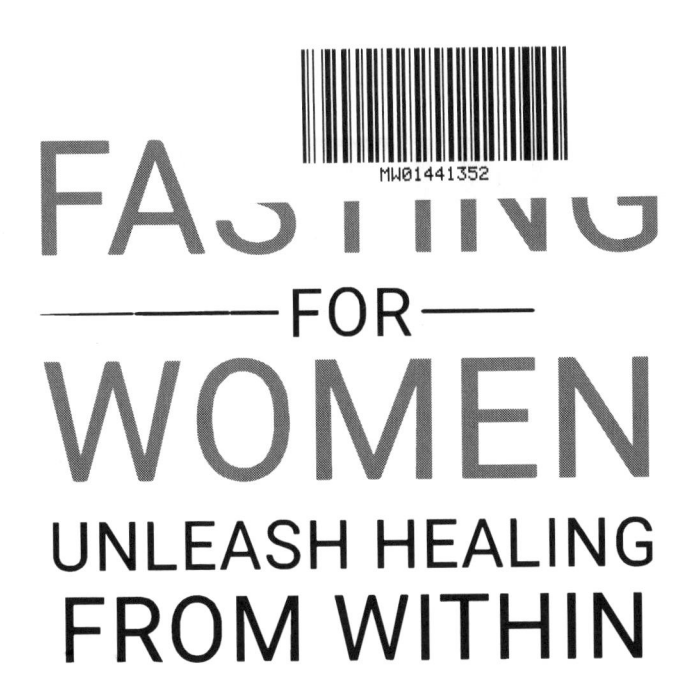

UNLEASH HEALING FROM WITHIN

A WOMAN'S GUIDE TO NATURAL WELLNESS AND WEIGHT MASTERY

AMY C HURT

Table of Contents

My Personal Message to You v
    My Soapbox vii

Chapter 1: Understanding Fasting 01
    What is Fasting? 02
    Types of Fasting 05
    Historical Significance of Fasting 06
    Benefits of Fasting 09
    Weight Management and Fasting 10
    Cognitive Health and Fasting 15
    Fasting and Hunger 19
    Debunking Common Myths and
    Misconceptions 21
    Setting Intentions for Exploring Fasting 24

Chapter 2: Types of Fasting 31
    Intermittent Fasting 34
    Eat-Stop-Eat 46
    Fast Mimicking or 5:2 Eating Plan 52
    Extended Fasting 54
    Liquid and Dry Fasting 59
    Religious and Spiritual Fasting 62

Chapter 3: Mental & Emotional Preparation 69
    Your 'Why' is Your Compass: A Gentle
    Nudge Towards Finding Your True North 70
    Creating a Vision Board: A Proactive
    Strategy for Success 74

Expectations VS Reality 77
Tips for Hunger Management 82
The Grand Vision: Keeping Your Eyes on
the Prize 88

Chapter 4: Fasting Made Easier 93
Hunger Hacks: Worth A Try 93
Nourishing Foods for Breaking Fast 97
Exercise and Movement During Fasting 100
Adapting Fasting to Energy Levels 103
Flexibility Over Rigidity 104
The Psychological Aspect 105
When to Pause or Modify Fasting Practice 105
Fasting and Your Lifestyle 107
Social Events and Fasting 109
Fasting and Nutrition 111
Sustainability and Enrichment 113

Sample Fasting Schedules 117

Getting Started Methods 119
Becoming Metabolically Flexible 119
Intermittent Fasting Plan 122

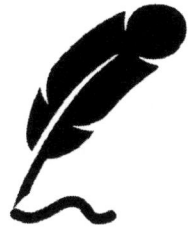

My Personal Message to You

Before we get deeply involved, I wanted to make my introductions: I'm neither a dietitian with a stack of certifications nor a doctor with a flair for fancy terms. Rather, I'm an explorer, much like you, who stumbled upon fasting in its various forms as a compelling approach to weight loss, which then lead me down the path toward overall well-being. No more counting calories, cryptic plans, or complex schedules; just a method anchored in simplicity and adaptability… AND is firmly backed by science, not someone trying to sell you the next best thing.

I've spent my entire adult life battling my weight and in my 30s my body tossed an auto-immune disease into the mix… that was less than helpful! I've tried every diet, exercise program, shake, smoothie, and supplement you can think of and all I got for it was an empty wallet. Nothing I tried moved the needle in the right direction for me. I had started to accept that "this is it" and I may as well go buy bigger jeans and pony up the exorbitant amounts of money for medications because I'm tired of fighting.

Then I came across intermittent fasting. I was intrigued and started digging in for a better understanding. The more I read, the more I felt this could possibly be the game changer I had been looking for in my life. The more I studied about fasting in its various forms, the more my mindset evolved from hoping to lose a few pounds to working toward my best health and wellbeing in years. Yes, please! I'm a Certified Life Coach, an EMT-IV, and a Corporate Environmental, Health, Safety and Security Manager by profession so this research and working to optimize my health fit right into my wheelhouse. I was pumped and couldn't wait to learn more!

After marching down this path for a period adequate to see the profound changes my body has gone through, I'm having this mind-blowing revelation that OUR BODIES HEAL THEMSELVES if we set ourselves up to allow that to happen. Once that lightbulb came on, I totally jumped into the deep end of the pool. I cannot express deeply enough: YOUR BODY IS A MIRACLE. Your body is meant to work WITH NATURE. We all just need a bit of understanding and a perspective adjustment to see what we need to be doing, or not doing, to allow the miracle that we live in to be the best it can be. Our bodies are absolutely amazing! Let's dig in…

My Personal Message to You

My Soapbox

During the time I have spent focusing on good health, good food, and making good (or at least better) lifestyle choices, the more disappointed I have become with the current state of things in the United States food space as a general statement. I could probably write an entire book on this subject alone… but I'll just give you my condensed version. I'm doing this before digging into fasting so that it might widen your perspective and allow you to see fasting and the contents of this book as a component of a healthy lifestyle. This is not an instant fix for a singular issue. This is a lifestyle choice on a path to a healthier you.

We don't have a healthcare system in the US, we have a SICK care system. Traditional medicine seeks to provide a pill for what ails us rather than teach us how to PREVENT illnesses. We've all been trained to believe this is a linear process. You experience XYZ symptoms, go to the doctor, get ABC pill(s) prescribed… which we believe will FIX the problem. The entire system is driven by dollars, not good health. And the pills DON'T fix the problem most of the time. They may lessen a symptom but will probably add another symptom or five! This saddens me deeply. We've all gone through a pandemic together in the last few years and what we heard broadcasted over the air waves and TV screens was: Shelter in place, wear a mask, bathe in hand sanitizer and alcohol to kill all the germs, and wait on the miracle vaccine to arrive.

Instead, what we should have been hearing and seeing is how we can make small changes to improve our health and immunity…. Go outside and get your vitamin D from the sun, put your hands and feet in the dirt where you can benefit from the GOOD bacteria and organisms there, eat whole foods that are nutrient dense rather than deep fried processed food that has little to no nutritional content, and stop putting toxins in and on your body as much as you can! We should have all started learning to fast together during the pandemic rather than learning to be fearful of one another… who might sneeze, who touched the door handle, who to blame for the next bad thing. Viruses would not survive, or have a VERY hard time with it in a body that is in a fasted state… there is not a bunch of sugar in the blood for the virus to feed upon and multiply. The next time you get a virus of any kind, stop eating. You'll be amazed at how quickly it goes away!

Chemicals… this was another big hitter I had honestly not considered prior to this health journey. I'm a safety person by profession so I knew to wear protective gear when handling certain chemicals… but what about the chemicals in our laundry soap, lotions, shampoos, and even toothpaste! Seek cleaner, non-toxic alternatives for these products. Seek natural cleaners to use in your home. Use essential oils, herbs, and spices…. You will be very impressed by the expansive solutions these natural products can offer! Even for your lawncare… NO MORE ROUNDUP or chemicals on your garden plants!!!

My Personal Message to You ix

Of course, I'm not suggesting you throw out everything in your home you've spend hundreds of dollars to purchase. No. Rather, when it's time to purchase more of something, seek a cleaner, non-toxic version. You'll slowly improve your environment in this way without breaking the bank.

Supplements are ok if you ensure you are using clean ones, not those full of unwanted fillers. But, once again, we cannot supplement our way past a toxic environment or a terrible diet. Think clean here too!! Please do not buy your supplements at Walmart. No offense, but that's not where the good ones are sold! Avoid those with heavy metals, artificial colors and dyes, avoid taking pills you may be able to do without. Have a headache? Try peppermint oil on your temples and the base of your skull at your neckline. Try meditation and breath work. Try taking a walk. Try something natural before you reach for the bottle of tablets.

We should begin to look upstream of our health concerns rather than seek a pill for each thing. This took me a LONG TIME to realize, but now I see it all too clearly. What is provided in our stores, advertised in every possible media, and even reported to us on the news is all driven by profit. Step back from what you hear and see and think for yourself about what you are about to 'consume' whether it's food, a podcast, a tv show, or a supplement. Is it good for you? Does it add value to your life? We all need positive energy, whole and nutritious food, and less stress to live healthier lives.

Diving into fasting made me realize there are so many things I could do to improve my health that didn't cost a thing!! Adopting a fasting lifestyle actually made the cost of my groceries go down! Choosing whole foods around the outside of the grocery store cost less than the processed junk in the bags and boxes even when I buy organic! Going outside and spending time in nature and soaking in a bit of sunshine is free! Taking a walk is free! Connecting with friends and sharing positive energy is free! Getting a hit of 'happy chemicals' in my brain by petting my dog or hugging a friend is FREE.

This journey has been truly transformative for me in so many ways, and I hope it is for you too! Please read this book knowing that YOU are in the driver's seat of your health. YOU can absolutely change your health for the better. And you are not stuck with any single 'solution.' You are free to explore a lifestyle of using various fasting methods that work for you.

With all of that said, I send you my deepest love and encouragement from my soul to yours. Give yourself grace and embark upon this knowing you are giving yourself the gift of better health. Step into this one foot at a time by making small sustainable changes. Come at this from a place of self-love and respect and you'll succeed beyond your wildest expectations. Now let's do this!

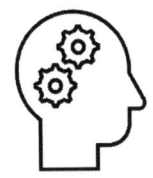

Chapter 1

Understanding Fasting

Ever thought about not eating for a bit? And no, I don't mean that time you slept in and missed breakfast. Intermittent fasting might sound like a trend where you play hide-and-seek with your food. But in reality, it's more of a method to tune into your body's natural rhythms.

If diets were movie sequels, I'd have seen them all: "Calorie Counting 1", "Trendy Diet 2: The Carb Returns", and "Detox Smoothies: The Green Revenge". You get the picture. Yet, amidst this blockbuster mayhem, I stumbled on intermittent fasting, and it felt like the classic film that wins all the awards.

In this guide, we'll navigate the ins and outs of this 'scheduled eating'. We'll sift through the science without making you feel like you're back in high school biology and highlight the multitude of benefits. Hint: it's not about going to bed dreaming of a sandwich, but more about aligning with a routine that complements your lifestyle.

Using the knowledge I've gathered, I aim to present a clear, and hopefully a tad entertaining, roadmap for you to follow on your journey. Whether you're aiming to shed some lingering weight, invigorate your energy levels, or cultivate a healthier relationship with food, intermittent fasting might just be the ticket.

The best part? It's not a one-size-fits-all. It's tailored to fit the suit that is your life. I'm here to help you measure it correctly, perhaps with a chuckle or two to ease the process. With a happy and hopeful heart, let's get with it!

What is Fasting?

Fasting, in its simplest form, is the voluntary abstention from food for a specific period. It's not a newfangled trend or a radical dieting technique; it's a practice that has been a part of human culture and evolution for centuries. In fact, our ancestors often had to fast involuntarily due to food scarcity, and our bodies have evolved to adapt to periods of fasting.

I know what you might be thinking: "Why on earth would anyone willingly skip meals?" It's a valid question, and one I had myself when I first heard about fasting.

Understanding Fasting

The primary reason people choose to fast, and why it has gained so much attention in recent years, is because of its potential health benefits. Fasting isn't just about cutting calories; it's about allowing your body time to rest, repair, and rejuvenate. When you fast, several physiological changes occur that can lead to improved health and well-being.

Here are some of the key benefits of fasting that we'll explore in detail throughout this book:

1. **Weight Management:** Fasting can be an effective tool for weight loss. By restricting the window of time in which you eat, you naturally consume fewer calories, leading to weight loss. Additionally, fasting may help regulate hormones involved in appetite and metabolism, among other things.

2. **Improved Insulin Sensitivity:** Fasting can enhance your body's sensitivity to insulin, reducing the risk of type 2 diabetes. It helps lower blood sugar levels and can even help those with diabetes manage their condition more effectively.

3. **Cellular Autophagy:** Fasting triggers a process called autophagy (pronounced aw-taw-fa-gy), where your cells remove damaged components and recycle them. This can have a profound impact on cellular health and longevity. It is literally cellular maintenance that you can control! What? I know!! We will learn that fasting actually triggers this process, so cool!

4. **Enhanced Brain Function:** Studies suggest that fasting may improve cognitive function, protect the brain from age-related diseases, and boost mental clarity and focus. Are you kidding? Who doesn't want that!?!?

5. **Longevity:** While more research is needed, fasting has been associated with extended lifespan in certain animal studies. It's an exciting area of research with potential implications for human longevity.

6. **Simplified Eating:** Fasting can simplify your relationship with food. Instead of constantly worrying about what to eat or when to eat, fasting can free up mental energy and promote a more intuitive approach to eating. It can at last free you from the monotonous calorie counting!! Free at last, free at last!!

7. **Gut repair:** Fasting is one of the most impactful things one can do to repair gut issues. Many of us may not even realize just how bad the situation is in our gut until we start digging into what is causing uncomfortable symptoms… Leaky gut and gut dysbiosis or microbiome damage after antibiotics are all real and very common. When you allow your body to unleash its natural superpowers, amazing healing takes place.

And much more … memory issues and accelerated aging? Fasting is for you! Suffering with an autoimmune disease? Fasting is for you! Struggling with depression and anxiety? Fasting is for you!

That said, it's important to note that fasting isn't a magic bullet, and it's not suitable for everyone all the time. There are various fasting methods, and what works for one person may not work for another. Your age, current health status, and lifestyle all play a role in determining the right approach for you. We should also know it's GOOD to change things up and not pick one thing, one way of eating, and do that every day for ever. Your life is not like that, why should your way of eating be? So, let's talk about fasting varieties and what might work for you.

Types of Fasting

Fasting is a practice that involves voluntarily abstaining from food for a specified duration. It's important to note that fasting isn't synonymous with starvation. I repeat, it is NOT starvation. While starvation is often involuntary and harmful, fasting is a controlled and deliberate choice that can have numerous health benefits and you are in complete control.

People turn to fasting for various reasons, and it's essential to understand the motivations behind this practice. Fasting is a versatile tool that can help with weight management, and so many other conditions and challenges. By exploring your "why," you can better tailor your fasting approach to aim directly for your unique goals.

Fasting can take different forms, allowing individuals to choose a method that aligns with their lifestyle and preferences. Common fasting methods include:

- **Time-Restricted Eating:** This approach restricts eating to a specific window of time each day. One chooses the number of fasting hours, and the remainder is the eating window.

- **Extended Fasting:** Extended fasting involves fasting for more extended periods, typically more than 24 hours.

- **Alternate-Day Fasting:** This method alternates between days of regular eating and days of fasting.

Exploring these methods allows individuals to find the fasting approach that best suits their goals and lifestyle. We'll go into detail about this in chapter 2.

Historical Significance of Fasting

Fasting holds a profound historical and cultural significance in societies around the world. Its roots extend deep into the annals of human history, where it has played diverse roles across various domains.

Religious Practices: One of the most prominent aspects of fasting's historical significance is its association with religious traditions. In Christianity, fasting during Lent commemorates Jesus's 40 days of fasting in the wilderness. Muslims observe fasting during

Ramadan as an act of worship and self-discipline, marked by reflection, prayer, and community. Judaism incorporates fasting into the observance of Yom Kippur and other significant holidays. Fasting is also prevalent in Hinduism, Buddhism, and other religions, each with its own spiritual purpose and significance.

Health and Healing Traditions: Fasting has been an integral part of traditional medicine systems. Ayurveda, in India, and Traditional Chinese Medicine have both employed fasting as a means to promote the body's self-healing mechanisms and restore balance to vital energies. Additionally, many ancient civilizations recognized fasting as a method to facilitate physical and spiritual well-being.

Ancient Philosophers and Philosophical Movements: Fasting was explored by numerous philosophers and philosophical movements. Pythagoras, Plato, and the Stoics viewed fasting as a way to enhance mental clarity, discipline, and self-control. They believed it could aid in achieving a deeper understanding of the self and the world. I tend to agree.

Political and Social Movements: Fasting has also been employed as a form of political protest and social advocacy. Mahatma Gandhi famously used hunger strikes as a nonviolent means to draw attention to social injustices and push for political change. Fasting, in this context, became a powerful tool for individuals to effect transformative societal shifts.

Cleansing and Detoxification: Many ancient cultures embraced fasting as a means to purify the body and cleanse it of impurities. Fasting rituals were associated with physical and spiritual purification, allowing individuals to seek harmony and clarity within themselves. Fasting can, and is, used for detox today as well.

Cultural Traditions: Fasting is integrated into various cultural traditions. For instance, some Native American tribes incorporate fasting into vision quests, where individuals seek spiritual guidance and revelation through this practice. Such traditions reflect fasting's connection to cultural identity and spiritual growth.

Seasonal and Agricultural Significance: In agrarian societies, fasting often had seasonal and agricultural connotations. It could be a way to conserve food during periods of scarcity or to align with agricultural cycles, reflecting the close connection between fasting and the rhythms of nature.

These historical examples collectively underscore fasting's multifaceted role throughout human history. Beyond its physical aspects, fasting has been a conduit for spirituality, discipline, self-discovery, and even political and social change. Understanding this rich historical context enhances our appreciation of fasting as a practice deeply intertwined with the tapestry of human civilization.

Understanding Fasting

Benefits of Fasting

Fasting, an ancient practice with a contemporary twist, holds the key to a plethora of health benefits that go beyond the scale. In this section, we'll journey through the remarkable advantages of fasting, exploring how it can transform not just your body, but your entire approach to well-being.

From weight management to enhanced mental clarity and even the potential for a longer, healthier life, fasting has more to offer than meets the eye. Let's discuss these incredible benefits that have captivated the curiosity of health enthusiasts and scientists alike.

Disclaimer time… please note that I am not a physician and this book, and its contents are not meant to be medical advice on treating medical conditions. Please confer with your doctor on a treatment plan and diet that is right for you! Ok… and now we can continue ☺

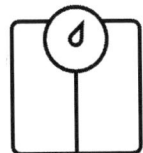

Weight Management and Fasting

Losing weight doesn't have to be complicated, and fasting offers a straightforward approach to achieving your weight loss goals. It's about using your body's natural abilities to burn fat for energy, making weight loss more manageable and sustainable. This method can be quite liberating if you are like me and have tried so many complicated methods and approaches in the past. Fasting keeps it simple and allows you to be in total control! I LOVE that!

The Science Behind Fasting and Weight Loss

Understanding how fasting aids in weight loss begins with the science behind it. When you fast, your body enters a state known as ketosis. During ketosis, your body switches from primarily using glucose (sugar) for energy to burning fat. This shift allows you to tap into your fat stores, which is precisely what you want when you're looking to shed extra pounds. Importantly, fasting helps preserve your muscle mass, so you're not losing important lean tissue along with fat.

There are not many people out there that have not yet heard of the Keto Diet. This is a way of eating that keeps the body in a state of fat burn rather than depending upon carbohydrates for energy. If weight loss is your primary goal, which it is in the beginning for many, combining fasting with a keto-style of eating can be unbelievably powerful! We'll dig into this a bit more in a bit.

Understanding Fasting 11

Appetite Control and Fasting

Contrary to what you might expect, fasting doesn't necessarily lead to extreme hunger. Many people find that fasting helps them better regulate their appetite. Over time, fasting can reduce cravings and promote a more balanced relationship with food. This improved appetite control can be a game-changer in weight management. Don't worry, I'll give you some 'hacks' to get you over the hump when you're getting started.

Sustainable Weight Management

Fasting isn't just about losing weight temporarily; it's a sustainable approach to weight management. By incorporating fasting into your lifestyle, you not only shed excess weight but also develop healthier eating habits. It's about achieving your weight loss goals and maintaining them for the long run, rather than going on and off diets. For me, this was the liberation I was looking for. I no longer count things, I don't weigh things, I don't track macros, I simply eat real food and my body takes care of the rest! Hallelujah!!!!

Diabetes and Fasting

Living with diabetes often involves meticulous attention to diet, medication, and lifestyle to maintain stable blood sugar levels. However, there's a promising approach that has captured the interest of both medical professionals and individuals with diabetes - fasting. In this section, we'll explore how fasting can become a potent ally in the battle to regulate blood sugar, enhance insulin sensitivity, and transform the management of diabetes.

Balancing Blood Sugar Through Fasting

At the heart of diabetes management is the challenge of keeping blood sugar levels in check. Fasting offers a unique perspective on achieving this balance. While it's not a universal solution, incorporating fasting into your routine can present a novel strategy for managing blood sugar levels effectively.

Science Behind the Connection

Understanding the synergy between fasting and diabetes management requires delving into the scientific principles at play. During fasting, the body undergoes notable changes that can positively impact insulin sensitivity and blood sugar regulation. This understanding forms the foundation for the potential benefits of fasting for individuals with diabetes.

Enhancing Insulin Sensitivity

A pivotal aspect of diabetes is the body's ability to respond to insulin. Fasting can play a crucial role in enhancing insulin sensitivity - the capacity of cells to effectively utilize insulin. By improving insulin sensitivity, fasting has the potential to facilitate better blood sugar control and reduce the reliance on external interventions.

Transforming the Diabetes Paradigm

Fasting is not a one-size-fits-all solution and must be approached with caution, particularly for those with diabetes. However, when executed under professional guidance, it can offer a fresh perspective on diabetes management. Fasting doesn't equate to deprivation; rather, it empowers individuals to reclaim control over their health. By exploring the science, strategies, and possibilities of fasting, individuals with diabetes can tap into a potent tool for blood sugar control and overall well-being.

Cardiovascular Disorders and Fasting

Our heart is the hardest-working muscle in our body, and maintaining its health is crucial for overall well-being. Emerging research suggests that fasting can be a powerful ally in supporting cardiovascular health. Let's explore the science behind this connection in a simplified way that my brain, and yours too, can wrap around.

The Cardiovascular System

First, let's briefly understand the cardiovascular system. It consists of the heart and a network of blood vessels that carry oxygen and nutrients to every cell in our body. A healthy cardiovascular system is essential for maintaining optimal health. When the body starts losing nutrients or the ability to carry nutrients, things start to decline.

The Role of Cholesterol

You've probably heard of cholesterol - it's a fatty substance in our blood. There are two types: LDL (low-density lipoprotein) and HDL (high-density lipoprotein). LDL is often referred to as "bad" cholesterol because having high levels of it can increase the risk of cardiovascular diseases, like heart attacks and strokes. HDL, on the other hand, is known as "good" cholesterol because it helps remove LDL from the bloodstream.

Fasting and Cholesterol Levels

Now, here's where fasting comes in. Studies have shown that fasting can have a positive impact on our cholesterol levels, particularly reducing LDL cholesterol. When you fast, your body taps into its fat stores for energy, which can lead to a decrease in LDL cholesterol levels. Additionally, fasting can promote the production of HDL cholesterol, further protecting your heart. It's like a 'behind the curtain' thing happening we aren't even aware of until we go to the doctor and our blood test results are improved.

Blood Pressure and Fasting

High blood pressure (hypertension) is another significant risk factor for CVDs. Fasting has been found to help lower blood pressure levels. During fasting, your body's production of a hormone called norepinephrine decreases. This hormone narrows your blood vessels and raises blood pressure. By reducing

Understanding Fasting

norepinephrine, fasting can contribute to healthier blood pressure levels.

Inflammation and Oxidative Stress

Chronic inflammation and oxidative stress are two processes that can damage blood vessels and increase the risk of CVDs. Fasting has been shown to reduce markers of inflammation and oxidative stress in the body. This means that fasting may help protect your blood vessels from damage, promoting cardiovascular health.

Weight Management

Maintaining a healthy weight is essential for heart health. Fasting can aid in weight loss and weight management, which, in turn, reduces the strain on your heart. Excess weight is a risk factor for cardiovascular diseases, and by shedding pounds through fasting, you can lighten the load on your cardiovascular system.

Cognitive Health and Fasting

Our brain, the epicenter of intelligence and cognition, deserves special attention when it comes to health.

There's a growing body of research suggesting that fasting can have a profound impact on cognitive function. Let's explore the science behind this connection in a way that's both insightful and easy to digest... pun intended.

The Brain's Remarkable Complexity

To understand how fasting influences cognitive health, let's start with the basics. The human brain is an intricate network of billions of neurons, constantly communicating with each other. Cognitive health refers to the well-being of our mental processes, including memory, attention, problem-solving, and more. That's a terribly simplified description, but you get it, right?

The Brain's Energy Source

Our brains are energy-hungry organs, and they primarily rely on glucose (sugar) for fuel. But here's where fasting becomes intriguing. During fasting, when we're not eating, our body's glucose levels dip. To compensate, our bodies start to use an alternative energy source: ketones. Ketones are molecules produced when our bodies break down fat. And guess what? Our brains love ketones just as much as glucose, maybe more! Ketones are a super-fuel for our brain in so many ways.

Fasting and Brain-Derived Neurotrophic Factor (BDNF)

One of the key players in fasting's impact on the brain is Brain-Derived Neurotrophic Factor, or BDNF. Think of BDNF as brain fertilizer - it promotes the growth and maintenance of neurons. Studies have shown that fasting can boost BDNF levels, potentially enhancing brain function. This could translate to improved memory, focus, and overall cognitive performance.

Autophagy: Cellular Cleanup for a Sharper Mind

Fasting, after a certain point, also triggers a process called autophagy, which is like a spring cleaning for your brain cells. During autophagy, your cells remove damaged components and recycle them. This process helps maintain the health of brain cells and could play a role in preventing age-related cognitive decline. More and more studies are showing fasting to have positive impacts on age-related brain diseases like Alzheimer's and dementia. Autophagy is a necessary process that many of us have not given our bodies the appropriate environment and conditions to perform.

Stress Resistance and Cognitive Resilience

Fasting might make your brain more resilient to stress. Stress can take a toll on cognitive health, but fasting appears to promote the production of proteins that protect brain cells from stress-related damage. This can contribute to greater cognitive resilience and adaptability. If you consider that your brain will primarily be running on ketones as fuel rather than sugar, you can see where this sense of calm and stress resilience may come from.

Intermittent Fasting and Mental Clarity

Have you ever noticed that after a meal, you might feel a bit sluggish or less focused? That's because digestion requires energy, and your brain's energy supply temporarily shifts towards your digestive system. During fasting, this diversion of energy doesn't happen, allowing your brain to function at its peak. Many people report heightened focus and mental clarity during fasting periods. Additionally, once your body starts using ketones as brain fuel, your focus and clarity make a noticeable shift to the positive.

Aging, Brain Health, and Fasting

As we age, cognitive decline becomes a concern. Fasting may offer some protection against age-related brain diseases like Alzheimer's and Parkinson's. While research is ongoing, fasting's potential to reduce risk factors like inflammation and oxidative stress may contribute to maintaining brain health as we grow older. We require less calories as we grow older as well, so perhaps this is nature's intent. We eat when we need nourishment, then fast to allow self-healing. That makes perfect sense to me!!

Fasting and Hunger

Hunger is something we all feel, and it's a significant part of our daily lives. So, how does fasting affect hunger? Let's break it down.

When you fast, especially for a while without eating, your body's hunger hormone, called ghrelin, increases. This hormone tells your brain that it's time to eat. That's why you might feel hungry when you're fasting - your body's way of saying, "I need food!"

Starting fasting might make you feel even hungrier initially. Your body needs time to adjust to this new way of eating. But the good news is that this intense hunger usually doesn't last long.

The timing of your meals during fasting plays a big role in how hungry you feel. If you're doing something like time-restricted eating, where you only eat during certain hours, you might feel hungry leading up to your first meal. But as your body gets used to this schedule, your hunger tends to become more predictable and easier to manage.

Hunger isn't the same for everyone. It can change based on things like how fast your body burns calories, how active you are, and what you ate in your last meal. Some fasting methods, like intermittent fasting, might actually reduce your overall hunger because your body becomes better at using stored energy, including fat, during fasting times. This is sometimes referred to as becoming "fat adapted" and this allows your body to switch between using sugar and carbs as fuel to ketones as fuel without you even realizing it's happening. No pain, no discomfort, no screaming hunger, no…. just a smooth transition. The body is amazing!

It's also important to know the difference between hunger and appetite. Hunger is your body's way of telling you it needs food. Appetite is more about your desire to eat, which can be influenced by things like seeing or smelling delicious food, social situations, or emotions. Fasting can help you become more aware of true hunger signals versus just wanting to eat for other reasons. I have found this to be true for me in many ways. I found that I munched out of boredom quite often and I also had a tendency to use food as a feel-good trigger when I was upset somehow. A 'state changer,' if you will. Now, I tend to choose going for a short walk or do some breathing exercises instead.

Lastly, staying hydrated during fasting can help with hunger. Sometimes, what feels like hunger is actually thirst. Drinking water or other non-caloric beverages can help ease this sensation. I find it beneficial to add a pinch of pink sea salt and a squeeze of lemon to my water. I always exceed my water intake goal for the day without having to force it in.

In summary, fasting can affect hunger by increasing the hunger hormone initially, but as your body adjusts, hunger usually becomes more manageable. How you time your meals during fasting matters, and everyone experiences hunger differently. Understanding the difference between hunger and appetite is key, and staying hydrated can help you feel less hungry during fasting.

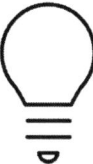

Debunking Common Myths and Misconceptions

Imagine if there was a single practice that promised weight loss, improved health, and increased vitality, all while allowing you to enjoy your favorite foods without guilt. It sounds like a dream, doesn't it? Yet, as with any trend that gains momentum, fasting has become a subject of myths and misconceptions that can cloud the truth behind its potential benefits.

In this section, we're stepping into the realm of myth-busting, where we'll separate fact from fiction and reveal the science-backed reality of fasting. As we journey through the most common misconceptions surrounding fasting, you'll discover that this ancient practice holds a world of promise, but it's crucial to navigate it armed with accurate information.

From the idea that fasting slows down your metabolism to the misconception that it's only meant for shedding pounds, we're here to dismantle these myths one by one. So, fasten your seatbelt—pun intended—as we embark on a journey to debunk these myths and uncover the genuine power of fasting for your health and well-being.

Ready to learn about the truth? Let's get it!

Myth 1: Fasting Slows Down Metabolism

Fact: Fasting does not necessarily slow down metabolism. In fact, some studies suggest that short-term fasting can boost metabolic rate. When you fast, your body may become more efficient at burning fat for energy, which can potentially enhance metabolic function. However, it's essential to approach fasting with a balanced and well-structured plan to maintain a healthy metabolism.

Myth 2: Fasting Leads to Muscle Loss

Fact: Properly executed fasting does not lead to significant muscle loss. When you fast, your body initially uses stored glycogen for energy. Once glycogen is depleted, it turns to fat stores for fuel while preserving lean muscle mass. In some cases, fasting may even help preserve muscle by promoting the release of growth hormones.

Myth 3: Fasting Causes Extreme Hunger

Fact: While you may experience hunger initially when you begin fasting, it typically diminishes over time. Fasting can actually help regulate appetite by reducing the production of the hunger hormone ghrelin. Many people find that fasting can improve their hunger control and make it easier to maintain a healthy eating pattern.

Myth 4: Fasting Is Only for Weight Loss

Fact: While fasting can be an effective tool for weight management, it offers a wide range of health benefits beyond weight loss. These benefits include improved insulin sensitivity, enhanced cognitive function, cellular autophagy (a cellular cleaning process), and potential longevity benefits. Fasting is a holistic approach to health that extends beyond the number on the scale.

Myth 5: Fasting Is Unsafe or Unhealthy

Fact: Fasting can be safe and healthy when done correctly. It's essential to approach fasting with knowledge and mindfulness. Always consult with a healthcare professional before starting a fasting regimen, especially if you have underlying health conditions or are taking medication. Fasting may not be suitable for everyone, but for many individuals, it can be a safe and effective practice when guided by evidence-based recommendations.

Myth 6: Fasting Is Extreme and Difficult to Sustain

Fact: Fasting doesn't have to be extreme or difficult to sustain. There are various fasting methods to choose from, allowing you to find an approach that fits your lifestyle and comfort level. Time-restricted eating, intermittent fasting, and gradual fasting protocols can be adapted to suit your preferences, making fasting a flexible and sustainable practice.

Myth 7: Fasting Is a Quick Fix for Health Issues

Fact: Fasting is not a quick fix, and it's essential to approach it as a long-term lifestyle choice. While it can yield positive health results, sustainable health improvements typically require consistency and a holistic approach that includes a balanced diet, regular physical activity, and other healthy habits.

By dispelling these common myths and misconceptions, you'll gain a more accurate understanding of fasting as a practice that, when approached thoughtfully and with knowledge, can offer a range of potential health benefits. Again, I recommend consulting with a healthcare professional before making significant changes to your diet or lifestyle, especially if you have underlying health concerns.

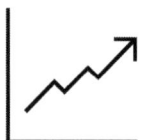

Setting Intentions for Exploring Fasting

Setting intentions for exploring fasting is a crucial step in preparing for your fasting journey. This involves

Understanding Fasting 25

establishing clear goals and a strong sense of purpose before you begin fasting. Here's a more detailed explanation:

Before you start fasting, it's essential to have a clear understanding of why you want to incorporate fasting into your lifestyle. This process involves:

1. **Identifying Your Goals**: Begin by identifying your specific objectives and goals for fasting. These goals can vary widely from person to person and may include weight loss, improved energy levels, better blood sugar control, mental clarity, or enhanced overall health. My personal goals were to drop a few pounds, feel better overall, and to overcome my autoimmune disease, rheumatoid arthritis.

2. **Defining Your Motivation:** Explore the underlying reasons driving your interest in fasting. Are you looking to feel more confident in your body, manage a health condition, or simply explore a new approach to wellness? Understanding your motivations will help you stay committed to your fasting practice. This is your 'true north' and can definitely help you stay on track when you have your mindset established. I like to say that I don't need motivation, I only need momentum moving forward.

3. **Creating a Personalized Plan:** Based on your goals and motivations, create a personalized fasting plan that aligns with your lifestyle and

preferences. Choose the fasting method that best suits your objectives, whether it's time-restricted eating, intermittent fasting, or another approach.

4. **Establishing a Timeline:** Set a clear timeline for your fasting journey. Determine the duration and frequency of your fasting periods and decide whether you want to start with shorter fasts and gradually increase the duration as you become more comfortable, or are you going to pick a method and stay the course? I find it works best for me personally to switch between intermittent fasting and no fasting, then mixing a longer fast into the mix every 6 to 8 weeks or so. Your plan will probably look different based upon your needs and lifestyle.

5. **Measuring Success:** Establish metrics for measuring your progress and success. Whether it's tracking changes in your weight, energy levels, blood sugar, or any other relevant indicators, having measurable goals will help you stay motivated and monitor your fasting's impact. This is a big one for me. We all like instant gratification so being able to SEE a tangible change is a huge driver to keep going. That said, DO NOT WEIGH IN DAILY. I repeat, don't weigh every day as this could send your day in the wrong direction if you don't see the result you expect.

   Many, like me, have a goal of dropping some weight. Rather than tracking progress with this solely by the number on the scales, I recommend taking body measurements. You'll really be pleased with your progress when you can see measurable results in so many places! Measure your waist, of course... no brainer there! Measure your biceps while holding your arms straight out to your side. Measure your thighs and measure around your hips. This one cracks me up because I feel like I'm measuring my butt as much as my hips! But when these numbers change, I'm so glad I took the time to do this!! This may be a good time to do 'before' photos as well. Again, when a side-by-side comparison reveals your progress, you'll be super pleased!

6. **Building a Support System:** Share your fasting goals with friends, family, or a supportive community. Having a support system can provide encouragement, accountability, and valuable insights as you navigate your fasting journey. Even better is if you have a friend or family member who goes WITH you on this journey. My husband and I are on the same eating plan which greatly simplifies grocery shopping, cooking, snack choices, and so on. Keeping two separate meal plans going is a very time-consuming thing and I'm grateful I no longer need to do that! Thanks, babe! I also have a number of friends and family that are embarking on their own journey as well. We may not all be going at the same pace or shooting for the same end goal... but we love to celebrate one another's successes and lift each other up.

7. **Staying Committed:** Remind yourself of your intentions regularly. Keep a journal or note

your goals in a visible place to stay focused and motivated. Celebrate your achievements along the way, no matter how small they may seem. Post yourself a note by the coffee pot or on the fridge door. I write in dry-ease marker on the glass wall in front of my desk. A little motivational quote here and there never hurts.

One tool I love for this is a journey board. You can use a small bulletin board, your refrigerator with some magnets, a page in a notebook or your journal, or any place you have where you can put some motivating things in a visible place. Cut out things that will push you to keep going. A palm tree to remind you of the vacation you want to take this summer (and look good in a swimsuit.) A super cute outfit you will reward yourself with when you reach a milestone goal should definitely go on the board! Motivational quotes or phrases are great to pin up... I like to keep adding to these and sometimes changing them out as I see fit. Make the board a part of the process to KEEP MOVING FORWARD.

Setting intentions is a vital step because it gives your fasting journey a sense of purpose and direction. When you know why you're fasting and what you hope to achieve, you'll be better equipped to stay committed, overcome challenges, and reap the rewards of this practice. Additionally, having a clear plan and goals will help you tailor your fasting approach to your unique needs and circumstances.

Understanding Fasting

Chapter Summary

Fasting, simply put, is taking a conscious break from eating. But it's more than just not eating; it's about giving the body a chance to refresh and rejuvenate.

When the body isn't constantly digesting food, it gets the opportunity to work on other tasks. It's like when you pause a busy workday to tidy up your desk. The body starts repairing cells, removing unwanted waste, and even uses stored fat for energy, which often leads to weight loss.

Interestingly, our brains also benefit from fasting. When we fast, the body begins to use fat as its primary source of energy, producing substances known as ketones. These ketones are a valuable energy source for the brain, which may help in enhancing brain health.

But fasting isn't just about the physical benefits. It also helps in understanding hunger better, recognizing the difference between eating out of habit and actual hunger. Overall, fasting offers an insightful journey into one's health, blending old wisdom with modern understanding.

References

1. Mattson, M. P., Longo, V. D., & Harvie, M. (2017). Impact of intermittent fasting on health and disease processes. *Ageing Research Reviews*, *39*, 46-58.

2. Horne, B. D., Muhlestein, J. B., & Anderson, J. L. (2015). Health effects of intermittent fasting: hormesis or harm? A systematic review. *The American Journal of Clinical Nutrition, 102*(2), 464-470.

3. Maslov, P. Z., Sabharwal, B., Ahmadi, A., Baliga, R., & Narula, J. (2022). Religious fasting and the vascular health. *Indian Heart Journal, 74*(4), 270-274.

4. Antoni, R., Johnston, K. L., Collins, A. L., & Robertson, M. D. (2017). Effects of intermittent fasting on glucose and lipid metabolism. *Proceedings of the Nutrition Society, 76*(3), 361-368.

5. Hatori, M., Vollmers, C., Zarrinpar, A., DiTacchio, L., Bushong, E., Gill, S., Leblanc, M., Chaix, A., Joens, M., Fitzpatrick, J., Ellisman, M., & Panda, S. (2012). Time-Restricted Feeding without Reducing Caloric Intake Prevents Metabolic Diseases in Mice Fed a High-Fat Diet. *Cell Metabolism, 15*(6), 848-860.

6. Tinsley, G. M., & La Bounty, P. M. (2015). Effects of intermittent fasting on body composition and clinical health markers in humans. *Nutrition Reviews, 73*(10), 661-674.

Chapter 2

Types of Fasting

Fasting might sound simple at first: you don't eat for a set amount of time. But there's much more to it than meets the eye. Over the years, different types of fasting methods have emerged, each with its specifics, benefits, and challenges. Let's unpack this world, one method at a time.

Historically, fasting has always been a part of human existence. Sometimes it was out of necessity when food was scarce. The cave-family couldn't just swing by the fridge for breakfast. In fact, they weren't even guaranteed a filling meal every day. It all depended upon the hunt, the fruits and vegetables in season, and so many other factors. This is key to our bodies having the amazing ability to adapt in times of restricted intake. Our bodies are very adept at fasting.

Other times, fasting was a conscious choice based on religious or cultural beliefs. Over time, as people realized the health benefits of fasting, it became less about survival and more about well-being… Which is where I stumbled into the conversation.

Today, with a combination of traditional practices and scientific research, we have several fasting methods to choose from. Some methods involve abstaining from food for a few hours every day, while others might involve fasting for an entire day or more. Each method has been developed considering different needs, lifestyles, and health goals.

Now, thanks to both ancient practices and modern science, there are several ways to fast. Each method has its characteristics, duration, and benefits. This chapter is dedicated to breaking down these methods. We'll discuss each one, looking into its background, its principles, and its potential benefits. The idea is to provide a comprehensive understanding of the broad range of options available in fasting.

Fasting is not just about not eating. It's a deliberate, structured approach to managing food intake in a way that offers health benefits. With various methods available, there's flexibility in how you can incorporate fasting into your life. As we move forward, we'll explore these methods in detail, helping you understand which might be the best fit for your needs and lifestyle, perhaps more than one!

Here are a few types of fasting:

1. **Intermittent Fasting (IF):** Cycling between eating and fasting intervals within a 24-hour span.

2. **Time-Restricted Eating (TRE):** A specific window for eating each day, with fasting in between. (16/8, 14/10)

3. **Alternate-Day Fasting:** Switching between days of normal eating and days of full or partial fasting.

4. **Extended Fasts:** Going without food for periods ranging from 48 hours to several days.

5. **The 5:2 Diet:** Five days of regular eating and two days of caloric restriction each week.

6. **Eat-Stop-Eat:** Incorporating one or two 24-hour fasts into your week.

7. **Religious and Spiritual Fasting:** Fasting methods rooted in religious practices, such as Ramadan, Yom Kippur, and Lent.

8. **Liquid Fasts:** Consuming only liquids like water, juice, or broth for a set period.

9. **Dry Fasting:** Abstaining from both food and water for a specific time, though this can be more challenging and requires extra caution.

Each of these methods offers unique experiences, challenges, and benefits. They range from the more lenient and flexible to the strict and demanding.

Remember, fasting isn't a one-size-fits-all journey. With this expansive palette of methods, you can tailor your fasting experience to align with your goals, body, and lifestyle.

Before we get deeper into these various forms of fasting, I also want to make it clear that you can utilize as many of these types of fasting as you like. In fact, it's encouraged to become metabolically flexible and not become overly militant about one particular method and cast out the rest. The more you go into and out of fasting cycles, your body will become more adept at switching into fat-burn mode. Eventually you'll be burning fat even in your sleep when conditions are right!!

Intermittent Fasting

Intermittent Fasting (IF) is a method that cycles between defined periods of eating and fasting. Unlike many dietary approaches that focus on what you eat, IF is all about when you eat. It's more of an eating pattern than a diet, and its flexibility has garnered widespread attention. Let's take a closer look.

16/8 Method

Imagine a day when you don't start eating until lunchtime and finish dinner by 8 pm. That's the 16/8 method. You're eating during an 8-hour window - say, between 12 pm and 8 pm. Outside of that, it's just water, tea, a black coffee, or other calorie-free beverages. This way, your body gets a 16-hour break from food. It's popular because many find it easy to follow. It essentially feels like skipping breakfast or having a late brunch. This is a great place to start!

Types of Fasting

The Science Behind the 16/8 Method

The 16/8 method, fondly known as the Lean-gains protocol, revolves around squeezing daily eating into an 8-hour window and fasting for the remaining 16 hours. But what's happening behind the scenes in our body during this cycle? Let's break it down.

Glucose and Insulin Dynamics

- **Glycogen Depletion:** When we eat, glucose is stored in the liver as glycogen. Typically, after 8-12 hours of fasting, these glycogen stores start to deplete. With the 16/8 approach, once you hit hour 12, you've got about 4 hours of fat burning.

- **Insulin Drop:** As you fast, and especially after your glycogen is depleted, your insulin levels drop, signaling the body to start burning stored fat. Lower insulin levels, combined with increased fat availability, allows for greater fat burning. This switch is a natural process called the metabolic switch. The transition from using glucose to fatty acids and ketone bodies as fuel results in enhanced fat burning.

Cellular Repair & Autophagy

- **Initiation of Autophagy:** The fasting window encourages cells to initiate autophagy, a cellular "clean-up" process. It's akin to the cell taking out its garbage. This involves the cells breaking down and metabolizing broken and dysfunctional proteins that build up inside cells over time. Higher rates of autophagy have potential anti-aging benefits and can protect against several diseases, including cancer and neurodegenerative disorders.

Hormonal Responses

- **Growth Hormone:** Fasting prompts the secretion of human growth hormone. Higher levels of this hormone facilitate fat metabolism, muscle growth, and are beneficial for overall health. In the context of the 16/8 method, these secretions can have an anabolic effect, which can help with muscle growth and recovery.

Appetite and Digestion

- **Ghrelin Dynamics:** Ghrelin, known as the "hunger hormone", may see a change in its secretion patterns. Over time, with a consistent eating window, the body may produce ghrelin predominantly in anticipation of the feeding window, potentially making the fasting window easier over time and reducing feelings of hunger. I found this to be true for me; my body began to predict the time I typically eat with a surge of Ghrelin.

- **Digestive System Rest:** By not constantly bombarding our digestive system with food, the gut gets a break. This might assist with better digestion during the feeding window, promoting more efficient nutrient absorption. The other, more amazing thing that happens here is gut lining repair. Your body will slowly repair a leaky gut as well as find it's groove with digestion and bathroom cycles. Some people settle into a daily pattern, others only go every two or sometimes three days. Either is fine, your body is unique and will find its optimal timing.

Improved Brain Health

- **BDNF Production:** Fasting can stimulate the production of brain-derived neurotrophic factor (BDNF). BDNF plays a vital role in cognitive function, mood regulation, and neural health. It supports the growth, survival, and function of neurons and is critical for learning, memory, and overall cognitive performance.

- Additionally, fasting enhances the process of **neurogenesis**, which involves creating new nerve cells in the brain. This process contributes to optimal mental functions like learning capacity and memory retention.

- Optimum fasting-induced BDNF secretion in humans is expected to occur after 12 hours of strict caloric limitation or fasting. Longer fasting periods may further enhance BDNF levels, but it's essential to find a balance that suits individual needs and health goals.

Heart Health

- **Positive Cardiovascular Markers:** With time, adherents of the 16/8 method often see improvements in heart health markers, including reduced inflammation, lower blood sugar and insulin levels, and improvements in blood pressure.

- Blood Sugar: IF can help regulate blood sugar levels by improving insulin sensitivity. This is crucial for preventing type 2 diabetes and reducing the risk of heart disease.

- Blood Pressure: Research shows that IF can lead to a decrease in blood pressure. Lower blood pressure is associated with a reduced risk of heart attacks and strokes.

- Cholesterol Levels: IF may improve lipid profiles by reducing total cholesterol and LDL (bad) cholesterol levels. Maintaining healthy cholesterol levels is essential for heart health.

- Triglycerides: High triglyceride levels are linked to an increased risk of heart disease. IF has been shown to lower triglyceride levels, promoting cardiovascular health.

- Strengthening Blood Vessels: Improved blood vessel function is another benefit of IF. Healthy blood vessels enhance circulation and reduce the risk of heart-related complications.

Who Can Try 16/8 Fasts?

The 16/8 fasting method is often considered one of the more approachable forms of intermittent fasting, making it a good fit for many. It's particularly attractive to beginners. For someone just dipping their toes into the world of fasting, the 16/8 method might feel like an extended version of what they already do every night. Essentially, the "fasting" period can usually include sleep, so it might just mean pushing breakfast a bit later or having dinner a bit earlier.

People with weight management goals might find this method beneficial. By shortening the eating window, there's potential to naturally reduce caloric intake, without the need for meticulous calorie counting. Over time, this can contribute to weight loss, especially if combined with a balanced diet, or even a keto diet, during the eating period.

If you're someone with an active lifestyle, the 16/8 method can slot in seamlessly. Regular exercisers can time their eating windows to surround workout times, ensuring they're consuming their nutrients when their bodies most demand them. This ensures that muscle recovery isn't compromised.

For those who appreciate a bit of routine in their lives, this method provides structure. With its consistent eating pattern, the 16/8 method can eliminate that late-night snacking or sporadic eating habits some people struggle with. It sets clear boundaries, which for some can simplify daily food decisions, making healthy eating choices a tad more straightforward.

Who Should Not Try 16/8 Fasts?

While the benefits are enticing, fasting, even in this moderate form, isn't for everyone. Pregnant or breastfeeding women, for example, have increased nutritional demands. Introducing a fasting routine during these periods may not be advisable, as it could limit necessary nutrient intake. Similarly, individuals with a history of eating disorders should approach fasting with caution. The structured eating windows, for some, can trigger unhealthy patterns or exacerbate existing conditions.

Furthermore, those with specific medical conditions, especially conditions like diabetes or those on certain medications, should tread carefully. The implications of fasting can vary and might interfere with medication schedules or how the body reacts to medicines. Likewise, as we age, our body's nutritional and metabolic needs shift. Older adults considering this method should consult with healthcare professionals to determine if it's the right fit. And of course, growing children and teenagers have unique dietary needs to support growth and development. Regular meals and snacks play a crucial role in their well-being.

14/10 Fasting

Now, for those who feel 16 hours might be a stretch, the 14/10 offers a softer start. You eat over 10 hours and fast for 14. This might mean you could have a late breakfast at 10 am and finish dinner by 8 pm. It's a little more flexible and gives an extended window for those mid-morning hunger pangs.

The Science Behind the 14/10 Fasting

Glycogen Depletion

When we eat, our body converts excess glucose into glycogen and stores it in our liver and muscles. Think of glycogen as your body's backup energy source. With a 14-hour fast, the body starts to tap into these glycogen stores after about 10 to 12 hours when the immediate glucose from the last meal is used up.

Fat Burning Mode

Once those glycogen stores start to dwindle, the body begins to search for alternative energy sources. It's like if your car ran out of gasoline and started using its reserves. In this case, the body starts converting stored fat into energy through a process called lipolysis. Then, the liver transforms these fats into ketones, an alternative fuel for the body.

Insulin Levels Drop

One of the significant hormones affected by fasting is insulin. After meals, insulin levels rise, helping our body store sugar and fat. But when fasting, especially during the prolonged periods of the 14/10 method, insulin secretion decreases. Lower insulin levels promote fat burning and have other potential benefits for metabolic health.

Autophagy

During extended periods without food, our cells initiate a process called autophagy. Picture it as the cells' housekeeping crew, tidying up and getting rid of old or dysfunctional cell components. This cleanup process is essential for cellular health and proper function.

Hormonal Adjustments

Apart from insulin, other hormones come into action. Norepinephrine (noradrenaline) levels rise, which can help boost metabolism and energy expenditure. There's also a boost in the growth hormone, essential for growth, metabolism, and muscle strength.

Brain Health

Even though the 14/10 method isn't as extended as some other fasting types, there's still potential for increased production of brain-derived neurotrophic factor (BDNF). BDNF supports the brain's neurons, potentially improving mood, focus, and cognitive function.

Gradual Adaptation

A 14/10 split can be a gentler introduction to fasting than more extended periods. The body starts to adapt to the fasting rhythm, becoming more efficient in switching between glucose and fat as its primary fuel source.

The 14/10 fasting method initiates several biological processes that can be beneficial for health. While it doesn't plunge as deeply into the fasting state as longer periods might, it still provides a balanced approach for those wanting to explore intermittent fasting without diving into longer fasting windows.

Who Can Try 14/10 Fasts?

The 14/10 fasting method, which involves 14 hours of fasting followed by a 10-hour eating window, offers a balanced approach to intermittent fasting. This balance can be particularly suitable for a variety of individuals, and here's why.

For those who are new to the world of intermittent fasting, the 14/10 method provides a less intimidating introduction. Starting with longer fasting periods can be a shock to the system, both mentally and physically. But with a 14-hour fast, one essentially extends the natural overnight fast by just a few hours. It's an opportunity to adjust to the sensation of fasting incrementally. This gentle initiation makes it more palatable and sustainable for beginners, helping them ease into the rhythm of fasting without feeling overwhelmed.

Then, there are the active individuals. For those who lead a physically demanding lifestyle, whether it's due to regular gym sessions, jogging, or even brisk walking, there's a need for a consistent source of energy. With a 10-hour window to consume food, these individuals can comfortably fit their meals in, ensuring they receive the necessary nutrients and calories. This ensures they're not left feeling fatigued or devoid of the energy required for their physical routines.

Busy professionals might also find the 14/10 method to be a perfect fit. The modern-day work schedule can be hectic, and not everyone is a breakfast person. Some might find it more convenient to start their day without the hassle of preparing a morning meal. Instead, they can focus on their tasks and then indulge in a hearty meal later in the day. This method can align seamlessly with their routines, allowing them to stay nourished without compromising on their professional commitments.

There are individuals who are consciously trying to curb late-night snacking habits. For them, having a set cut-off time in the evening can be beneficial. By knowing they have a specific window in which they can eat, it creates a structure, potentially reducing the chances of mindless snacking late into the night.

Lastly, those who have previously tried other fasting methods and found them too restrictive might find solace in the 14/10 approach. It offers flexibility, which can be the key for many when it comes to long-term adherence. The good thing about 14/10 method is that it can be adapted to fit various schedules, making it a versatile choice for a wide range of individuals.

Who Should Not Try 14/10 Fasting?

The 14/10 fasting method, involving 14 hours of fasting followed by a 10-hour eating window, might seem relatively moderate compared to more intense fasting protocols. However, it's essential to acknowledge that it might not be suitable for everyone. Several groups of individuals should exercise caution or avoid it altogether.

Firstly, individuals with certain medical conditions, particularly those related to blood sugar regulation like diabetes, might face complications. Extended periods without food can influence blood sugar levels. For someone dependent on insulin or other diabetes medications, this can pose risks. If blood sugar drops too low without timely food intake, it might lead to hypoglycemia, which can be dangerous.

Another group that should be cautious is individuals with a history of eating disorders. Intermittent fasting, even a relatively moderate approach like the 14/10 method, can potentially trigger negative patterns or unhealthy obsessions with food. It's crucial for these individuals to prioritize their mental well-being and consult with healthcare professionals if considering any fasting method.

Pregnant or breastfeeding women should also stay away of this fasting method. During pregnancy and lactation, the body's nutritional needs increase, and consistent nourishment becomes critical. Restricting the eating window might compromise the nutrient intake required for both the mother's health and the child's development.

Similarly, individuals who are underweight or have a high metabolism might find this method counterproductive. If someone is already struggling to maintain or gain weight, limiting their eating hours can further hinder their ability to consume enough calories throughout the day. This can exacerbate the risk of nutritional deficiencies and negatively impact overall health.

Lastly, those who engage in high-intensity workouts, especially early in the morning or late at night, might find the 14/10 method restrictive. Their bodies may require a quick refuel after rigorous exercise sessions, and a strict eating window might not always align with their workout schedules, potentially hampering recovery and muscle growth.

Eat-Stop-Eat

This is like hitting the pause button on eating. For a full 24 hours, once or twice a week, you don't consume any food. Just fluids. It might sound intense, and it can be a challenge, but some people find it a good way to reset their system occasionally. For instance, if you finish dinner at 7 pm on a Friday, you'll eat next at 7 pm on Saturday. Some also call this alternate day fasting and fast for 24 hours, then not, then fast, then not.

The Science Behind the Eat-Stop-Eat Fasting

The Eat-Stop-Eat approach is another form of intermittent fasting. Unlike daily time-restricted feeding methods such as 16/8 or 14/10, Eat-Stop-Eat involves a 24-hour fast once or twice a week. Let's explore the science behind what happens in the body during this fasting period.

Initiation (0-3 hours after last meal)

- **Blood Sugar Levels:** Shortly after eating, the body starts digesting and absorbing nutrients. During this period, insulin is released, aiding in the absorption of glucose from the bloodstream into the cells. As time progresses, blood sugar and insulin levels start to decline.

- **Digestive Process:** The body continues the process of digestion and absorption, breaking down carbohydrates into glucose, proteins into amino acids, and fats into fatty acids and glycerol.

Post-Absorptive Phase (3-24 hours)

- **Glycogen Breakdown:** As blood glucose levels drop, the body starts to use glycogen, a stored form of glucose found in the liver and muscles. Glycogen is broken down into glucose to provide energy.

- **Fat Mobilization:** Once glycogen stores begin to deplete, usually around the 12-hour mark, the body increases its reliance on fat as an energy source. Fatty acids are released from adipose tissue and used for energy, leading to fat breakdown.

- **Protein Conservation:** Contrary to popular belief, the body does not immediately begin to break down protein for energy. It first maximizes glycogen and fat utilization. However, if the fasting period were to continue for several days, the body could start utilizing proteins more significantly if fat became less readily available in the body.

- **Ketone Production:** As fasting continues and glucose becomes limited, the liver starts producing ketones from the breakdown of fats. Ketones can serve as an alternate energy source for many cells, including those in the brain.

Hormonal Changes

- **Decrease in Insulin:** With prolonged fasting, insulin levels drop further, promoting fat breakdown.

- **Increase in Norepinephrine:** This hormone can increase metabolic rate, ensuring the body maintains energy production during the fasting state.

- **Increase in Growth Hormone:** Growth hormone secretion spikes, which has various beneficial effects, including muscle preservation.

Cellular and Molecular Responses

- **Autophagy:** This is a cellular "clean-up" process. Old, damaged cells or cellular components are broken down and recycled. Extended fasting can boost autophagy, potentially providing benefits like disease prevention.

- **DNA Repair:** There is evidence to suggest that fasting can increase the body's repair mechanisms, including those acting on DNA. Your DNA expression can also change as a result of your dietary changes. For example, you may have had an allergy to a particular food that is no longer a problem after you've lived a fasting lifestyle for a period of time.

Cognitive and Mood Effects

Some people report heightened clarity and improved mood during extended fasts, which might be linked to the increased production of brain-derived neurotrophic factor (BDNF) or the use of ketones as brain fuel during fasting.

By the end of the 24-hour fast, the body will have made significant metabolic shifts. Glycogen stores may be low, fat utilization will be heightened, and there may be increased levels of ketones in the blood.

When breaking the fast, it's essential to reintroduce food gently, especially if one isn't used to a full 24-hour fast. I often break my fasts with a protein-rich liquid like bone broth. The state of 'fasting' is broken when insulin levels go up, not simply because you put food in your mouth. One could eat half of an avocado, which is primarily fat... good fat... and your body would stay in autophagy and in an overall 'fasted' state. If you choose to go in for a meal, a balanced meal with moderate protein and healthy fats is typically recommended to replenish the body. If you are consuming carbs, choose slow carbs like sweet potatoes and avoid processed foods, like white bread.

Who Can Try Eat-Stop-Eat Fasts?

The Eat-Stop-Eat fasting method, which revolves around a 24-hour fast once or twice a week, has caught the attention of many. While intriguing, its adaptability really depends on the individual. Generally, healthy adults without significant underlying medical issues can consider giving this method a whirl. Especially those who've dabbled with other intermittent fasting routines, like the 16/8 or 14/10, might find stepping into a full-day fast an enticing challenge.

The Eat-Stop-Eat method naturally reduces weekly caloric intake, which can lead to weight loss. This approach can be helpful for individuals looking to create a calorie deficit without actively counting calories every day. Then there are the metabolic health enthusiasts drawn by benefits like enhanced insulin sensitivity and improved fat mobilization. On the convenience front, for anyone bogged down by daily meal planning and prep, having a couple of days off can be quite liberating. It also offers flexibility for those with unpredictable schedules, allowing them to slot in their fasting days as per convenience.

However, a 24-hour fast isn't just a physical game; it's mental too. It demands a certain mindset, one that's comfortable with recognizing and understanding body signals, especially those hunger pangs, and possesses the grit to see it through. But, and it's an important but, it's not a one-size-fits-all. Individual circumstances, health situations, and a nod from healthcare professionals are paramount before embracing this or any significant dietary change.

Who Should Not Try Eat-Stop-Eat Fasts?

The Eat-Stop-Eat fasting method, involving a full 24-hour fast once or twice a week, can be beneficial for many, but it's not for everyone. This may become predictable, but I want to clearly address that there are circumstances in which this is not advised. Individuals with certain medical conditions, such as diabetes, low blood pressure, or a history of eating disorders, should approach this with caution.

Pregnant and breastfeeding women are typically advised to maintain a steady intake of nutrients for both their well-being and that of the baby. Then there are those undergoing high-intensity training or physically demanding jobs that may require greater nutritional intake. People on specific medication regimens, especially those that require food intake, should be wary. A day without food can alter the effectiveness or even cause side effects with certain medications.

Older adults, or any age for that matter, with a frail physique who might already be battling malnourishment or muscle wastage would certainly not be in a position to enter 24-hour fasts. And individuals prone to migraines or severe headaches might notice an uptick in frequency or intensity due to the stress of fasting. Fasting can sometimes trigger these episodes, especially if dehydration sets in.

Lastly, it's essential to consider one's mental and emotional state. People who experience extreme stress, anxiety, or depression might find that fasting exacerbates their emotional state. The lack of food can sometimes magnify feelings of anxiety or mood swings.

In any case, while intermittent fasting methods, including Eat-Stop-Eat, can offer various benefits, it's imperative to remember the individual nature of nutrition and health. What works wonders for one person might be detrimental to another. Always seek advice from healthcare professionals before undertaking significant changes to eating patterns.

Fast Mimicking or 5:2 Eating Plan

This one breaks the week into regular days and low-calorie days. For five days, eat as usual, no restrictions. On the other two days, you drastically reduce your intake, sticking to just 500-600 calories. This method is sometimes referred to as fast mimicking. It's not full fasting but significantly cuts down food intake. It gives a balance of freedom and structure. So, you could eat normally from Monday to Friday and then limit your intake on the weekends. Or, you could pick any two days of the week that suit you best.

How & Why it Works

This method does not cause the body to do wildly different things in comparison to the other methods of fasting previously discussed. I'll not test your patience by repeating in detail how all of this works.

We know the body uses glycogen stores in the liver as its main energy source until that is depleted. Then, once glycogen stores are depleted, the body transitions into fat-burning mode, called lipolysis, and it releases fatty acids and glycerol, which are further broken down to provide energy.

As the body continues to burn fat, the liver produces ketones, which act as an alternative energy source, especially for the brain. With intermittent fasting, especially short-term like 5:2, the body tends to prioritize fat for fuel and doesn't break down protein (muscles) until it's a last resort.

All the other benefits can still be realized with this eating style… increased insulin sensitivity, reduced inflammation, cellular repair called autophagy, hormone benefits, benefits to the heart, improved gut health, and so on. All of these things are activated in processes more like a dimmer switch rather than a definitive ON/OFF switch. Fast mimicking can be a great starting place or an alternative to put in the mix.

Extended Fasting

Extended fasting refers to any fast that exceeds a 24-hour period. While shorter fasts like intermittent fasting focus primarily on cycles of short-term calorie restriction, extended fasts take the concept a step further by significantly prolonging the fasting window. It's a more intense approach and is much less common than intermittent fasting methods, primarily because of the sheer commitment and potential risks involved.

How Does it Work?

Upon initiating an extended fast, the body goes through several metabolic phases, adapting to the absence of incoming food and adjusting its energy sources accordingly. The first 24 hours are crucial. During this time, glucose, the body's primary source of energy, is consumed, and levels in the bloodstream start to drop. This glucose originates from the carbohydrates consumed before the onset of the fast. In everyday conditions, the body predominantly relies on this easily accessible energy source.

As the glucose supply diminishes, the body searches for an alternative. Enter glycogen. Stored primarily in the liver, but also found in muscles, glycogen acts as the body's energy reserve. Think of it as an emergency backup generator. However, even this robust system has its limits. Within about 24 to 48 hours, these glycogen stores become depleted.

Types of Fasting

Now, with the primary and secondary energy sources used up, the body must get creative. This is where the truly remarkable aspect of extended fasting comes into play. The body transitions into a metabolic state known as ketosis. In this state, the liver begins to convert stored fat into ketones. Ketones, in turn, serve as an alternative fuel source for many organs, especially the brain. The brain is an energy-hungry organ, and while it can't utilize fat directly, it can indeed use ketones. This conversion from glucose dependency to ketone dependency is the hallmark of the ketogenic state, which is also the foundation of the ketogenic diet.

Beyond just ketosis, extended fasting sparks another fascinating process called autophagy. When food is absent for an extended period, the body starts a cellular clean-up process. It's like a recycling and waste management system at the cellular level. Damaged cells and proteins are broken down and either expelled or repurposed, potentially leading to improved cellular function and health.

But it's also worth noting that during extended fasting, especially when stretching to a couple of days or beyond, the body can start to tap into amino acids for energy. These amino acids are derived from the breakdown of proteins in the body, which could lead to muscle loss if not managed correctly.

Benefits and Limitations of Extended Fasting

Extended fasting is like hitting the reset button for your body, and here's why it's drawing attention:

- **Cellular Cleanup:** Extended fasting triggers autophagy. Imagine a crew inside your body that throws out the damaged parts and keeps things running smoothly. Autophagy does that at a cellular level.

- **Weight Management:** If you're looking to lose some weight, extended fasting might be an avenue. When you fast, your body turns to its stored fat for energy, which could lead to weight loss.

- **Blood Sugar Control:** Fasting might help your body handle sugar more effectively. When done correctly, it can make your body more responsive to insulin, which manages sugar levels.

- **Mental Boost:** Feeling foggy? Some individuals find that fasting clears up that fog, giving them better focus and sharper thinking, possibly because the body starts using alternative energy sources that are friendlier to the brain.

Considerations of Extended Fasting:

No practice is without its challenges, and extended fasting has a few things to consider:

- **Nutrient Shortage:** If you fast for too long too often, your body might miss out on essential nutrients. Like skipping oil changes in a car; eventually, your body might wear down. To manage this, you'll need to focus on nutrients when you are eating. Seek nutrient dense whole foods over foods that are processed. Additionally, an extended fast should not be undertaken too frequently. I recommend a 3 day fast quarterly. This kicks the body over into full-blown fat burning, ketosis, autophagy, gut repair, inflammation reduction, and so much more... but not too often!

- **Muscle Loss:** Along with fat, there's a chance your body might use a bit of muscle for energy. Not ideal if you're trying to maintain muscle mass. To avoid this, ensure you are eating adequate amounts of protein. If you are seeking fat loss, but not muscle loss, focus on a keto-style or carnivore-style of eating to ensure protein levels stay in an appropriate range. You can also initiate a process called mTOR. mTOR is an enzyme that controls biochemical resources, including amino acids, fat, ATP, glucose, and hormones. Essentially, mTOR measures your food intake and orchestrates the processes needed for building and growing tissues. After you break your fast, include 30 grams or more of protein in your meal to initiate mTOR and ensure you're maintaining appropriate, strong muscle mass.

- **Electrolyte Management:** Extended fasting might mess with the body's balance of essential minerals. To combat this, you'll need to replace the lost minerals in your beverage choices during the fast. Sodium, potassium, and magnesium are the primary focus when managing electrolyte levels. There are pre-measured supplement packs that can be added to your water to keep things simple. I'm a fan of LMNT brand as they keep the minerals balanced, add just enough flavor to the mix, and keep extra junk out. You can also use liquid minerals like Beam minerals or others. There are others out there as well, just be mindful of additives and preservatives your body doesn't actually need… or want!

- **Overeating Post-Fast:** After fasting, there could be a temptation to eat a lot to "make up" for the missed meals. This could counteract some fasting benefits. This is more of a mindset thing for me, but it can be physical hunger for some people as well. Two components come into play here. To address both the physical and mental aspect, you'll want to make this as easy on yourself as you can. To do this, break your fast with plenty of healthy fat in the mix, and you'll find yourself surprisingly satisfied with very little food. This could look like adding an avocado to the meal, or adding a good amount of coconut oil or olive oil to the meal. At this point you'll feel satisfied and happy with what you've accomplished.

- **Flavor profile resets:** Many find that after an extended fast, many flavors taste much more vibrant or even different entirely I like to break my fast with bone broth. And let me tell you… after not eating for three days, that is the most delicious thing I've ever tasted. Usually, the day following an extended fast will include a celebratory steak dinner complete with a ribeye anointed with rosemary butter and a side of mixed veggies. This is my favorite meal any time, but after a long fast it is simply indescribable. You'll see!

- **Not for Everyone:** Extended fasting isn't a one-size-fits-all. Some people, especially those with specific health issues, should steer clear or at least consult with a healthcare professional before trying it out.

Liquid and Dry Fasting

Liquid Fasting

Liquid fasting is essentially when one abstains from consuming solid foods and relies solely on liquids for nourishment. The idea is to give the digestive system a break from processing solids. This is my preferred method. I find this to be much easier for me personally and those I've worked with have had similar experiences. Each person will choose what works best for them, of course, but I will always stress that we need to listen to our body when stepping into new practices such as fasting.

How it Works

When engaged in a liquid fast, the consumption is limited to fluids. This can include water, herbal teas, broths, and in some versions, juices and smoothies. The emphasis is often on hydrating and detoxifying the body. Since the digestive system is not processing solid foods, it requires less energy, potentially allowing the body to focus on healing and regeneration.

Why Someone Might Choose This?

People opt for liquid fasting for various reasons:

- **Detoxification:** Clearing out toxins and giving the digestive system a break.

- **Weight Loss:** Even though you're consuming liquids, the calorie intake is typically reduced.

- **Medical or Health Reasons:** Sometimes, doctors might recommend a liquid diet before certain procedures.

- **Transition to or from a more intensive fast:** Liquid fasting can be a steppingstone for someone easing into or out of a more extended or strict fast. This can also be a great way to step into fasting while remaining somewhat 'normal' in your activities. But rather than ordering a meal when the family or business group goes out, order a healthy smoothie or just coffee or hot tea. You'll feel less like you're missing out if you have something to sip on.

Dry Fasting

This is considered one of the most intense fasting methods. Dry fasting entails refraining from consuming both food and liquids, including water, for a specified duration.

How it Works

When dry fasting, the body is devoid of any external sources of water or nutrition. This pushes it to seek hydration and nourishment from internal sources. The body might start to break down cells (including potentially harmful ones like damaged or diseased cells) for hydration and nutrition. It's a survival mode in the strictest sense.

Why Someone Might Choose This?

Dry fasting isn't as commonly practiced as other fasting types due to its intensity. However, those who advocate for it believe in its potential benefits:

- **Intense Detoxification:** The theory is that the body accelerates the removal of toxins when it doesn't have any external input.

- **Rapid Weight Loss:** Due to no intake and increased metabolic processes to sustain the body.

- **Spiritual or Religious Reasons:** Some cultures and religions use dry fasting as a form of spiritual cleansing or sacrifice.

However, it's crucial to note the potential risks of dry fasting. The body can become dehydrated, leading to a host of problems, from kidney issues to cognitive impairments. It's essential to approach this method with caution and under the guidance of a healthcare professional.

Religious and Spiritual Fasting

Fasting has deep roots in numerous religious and spiritual traditions. These fasts often carry a dual purpose: they address physical needs or desires while also fostering spiritual growth, reflection, or discipline. Here's a closer look at religious and spiritual fasting across various traditions:

Islam

Ramadan

During the holy month of Ramadan, Muslims around the world fast from dawn until sunset. This means abstaining from eating, drinking, smoking, and sexual relations during daylight hours. The fast is broken each day with a meal called iftar, which traditionally begins with eating dates.

Christianity

Lent

One of the most well-known Christian fasting periods is Lent, a 40-day season of reflection and preparation before Easter. Historically, many Christians abstain from certain foods (like meat) or pleasures during Lent. Fridays during this period often involve abstaining from eating meat.

Types of Fasting

Advent Fasting

Some Christian denominations observe fasting during Advent, the period leading up to Christmas.

Judaism

Yom Kippur

Known as the Day of Atonement, it's the holiest day in the Jewish calendar. Observant Jews fast for 25 hours, refraining from both food and drink.

Tisha B'Av

A day of mourning the destruction of both ancient Temples in Jerusalem. It's another 25-hour fast similar to Yom Kippur.

Hinduism

Ekadashi

Observed on the 11th day of each fortnight in the Hindu calendar. Devotees fast and abstain from certain foods, especially grains.

Navaratri

A nine-night festival where many devotees fast, consuming only fruits and dairy products.

Buddhism

In many Buddhist traditions, monks and nuns don't eat after noon, abstaining from food until the following sunrise. This practice is to ensure that they focus on their meditation and spiritual activities rather than the distractions of preparing and consuming meals.

Native American Traditions

Vision Quest

This is a rite of passage in some Native American cultures. The individual goes on a spiritual journey in a remote area, often involving fasting, to seek guidance or a vision.

Other Spiritual Movements

Fast for Peace

Inspired by Mahatma Gandhi's principles, many peace activists and spiritual leaders have adopted fasting as a nonviolent means of protest or to promote peace and understanding.

These examples merely scratch the surface. For many, fasting isn't just about abstaining from food or drink but also involves deep reflection, prayer, and a conscious connection to their spiritual or religious beliefs. Each tradition carries its unique nuances and significance, revealing the rich tapestry of human culture and spirituality.

Types of Fasting

Chapter Summary

At the core of modern fasting techniques is Intermittent Fasting, a cyclic eating pattern. It's less about what foods you eat and more about when you eat them. By alternating between eating and fasting periods, this approach brings the best of both worlds, offering flexibility and tangible health benefits.

The 16/8 Method is a popular form of intermittent fasting. With 16 hours of fasting followed by an 8-hour eating window, it often resembles skipping breakfast and avoiding those late-night nibbles. It's praised for its simplicity, and many claim it's almost like giving the body a nightly reset.

When we talk about the 14/10 Method, it's a softer landing into the world of fasting, especially for beginners. By eating over a 10-hour stretch and then fasting for 14 hours, it offers a balance that many find more manageable, particularly those not quite ready for the 16-hour fast.

Eat-Stop-Eat takes the concept a bit further. This method introduces a 24-hour fast, once or twice a week. It's like pressing a pause button on eating, allowing the body to dive deeper into its reserves for energy. Yet, with five unrestricted days, it doesn't feel overly demanding.

The 5:2 Diet offers another variation. Here, five days involve regular eating while the remaining two restrict calorie intake significantly, often to about 500-600 calories. It's like having two mini-detox days in the week, giving the body a break from continuous digestion.

When it comes to Extended Fasting (EF), we're in marathon territory. Spanning more than 48 hours, this method is for those who seek a deeper cleanse and reset. Given its length, it's crucial to be well-prepared and informed. Always consider professional advice before attempting such a long fast.

While liquid fasting permits the intake of fluids like water, broths, or juices, dry fasting is its more intense counterpart, barring all forms of liquid. These are advanced fasting techniques, and caution is of utmost importance.

Each method offers a unique approach, tailored to various needs and lifestyles. The key is understanding which one aligns best with individual health goals.

References

1. Gabel, K., Hoddy, K. K., Haggerty, N., Song, J., Kroeger, C. M., Trepanowski, J. F., Panda, S., & Varady, K. A. (2018). Effects of 8-hour time restricted feeding on body weight and metabolic disease risk factors in obese adults: A pilot study. *Nutrition and Healthy Aging*, 4(4), 345-353.

2. Cheng, C. W., Adams, G., Perin, L., Wei, M., Zhou, X., Lam, B., Da Sacco, S., Mirisola, M., Quinn, D., Dorff, T., Kopchick, J., & Longo, V. (2014). Prolonged Fasting Reduces IGF-1/PKA to Promote

Hematopoietic-Stem-Cell-Based Regeneration and Reverse Immunosuppression. *Cell Stem Cell*, 14(6), 810-823.

3. Anton, S. D., Moehl, K., Donahoo, W. T., Marosi, K., Lee, S. A., Mainous, A. G., Leeuwenburgh, C., & Mattson, M. P. (2017). Flipping the Metabolic Switch: Understanding and Applying the Health Benefits of Fasting. *Obesity*, 26(2), 254-268.

4. Trepanowski, J. F., & Bloomer, R. J. (2010). The impact of religious fasting on human health. *Nutrition Journal*, 9(1).

5. Effects of Intermittent Fasting on Health, Aging, and Disease. (2020). *New England Journal of Medicine*, 382(10), 978-978.

6. Harvie, M. N., Pegington, M., Mattson, M. P., Frystyk, J., Dillon, B., Evans, G., Cuzick, J., Jebb, S. A., Martin, B., Cutler, R. G., Son, T. G., Maudsley, S., Carlson, O. D., Egan, J. M., Flyvbjerg, A., & Howell, A. (2010). The effects of intermittent or continuous energy restriction on weight loss and metabolic disease risk markers: a randomized trial in young overweight women. *International Journal of Obesity*, 35(5), 714-727.

7. Varady, K. A., Bhutani, S., Church, E. C., & Klempel, M. C. (2009). Short-term modified alternate-day fasting: a novel dietary strategy for weight loss and cardioprotection in obese adults. *The American Journal of Clinical Nutrition*, 90(5), 1138-1143.

8. Patterson, R. E., & Sears, D. D. (2017). Metabolic Effects of Intermittent Fasting. *Annual Review of Nutrition, 37*(1), 371–393.

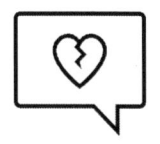

Chapter 3

Mental & Emotional Preparation

So, you've buckled up and set your mind to incorporate fasting. Good for you! But let's get one thing straight: this isn't your typical road trip. Oh no. This is less about scenic routes and more about dodging those pesky hunger potholes. And while you've got your foot on the gas, ready to ride, it's essential to remember that the journey of intermittent fasting isn't just a straight highway; it's more like a labyrinth of roundabouts, surprise detours, and occasional mirages of Grandma's apple pie.

You see, while your tummy's going, "Hey, where's breakfast?", your brain's diving deep into a nostalgic slideshow of every delicious meal you've ever had. Suddenly, that forgotten doughnut from three years ago seems as majestic as a unicorn. And that's where the real fun begins.

Fasting isn't just about resisting a bite of cake; it's about navigating the grand parade your brain hosts in honor of that cake. Now, wouldn't it be easier if we had a guide, perhaps sprinkled with a bit of humor, to help us maneuver these intricate emotional alleys?

Well, that's precisely what this section aims to offer. Think of it as a guide to understanding the quirks of our minds while fasting. I'll prepare you to face those unexpected emotional cravings and equip you with mental strategies to chuckle your way through them. So, fluff up your cushions, pour yourself a cup of your favorite beverage, and let's usher in a chapter where we learn to navigate the quirky, surprising, and utterly delightful maze of mental and emotional preparation for fasting. Because let's face it, a journey embarked on with a smile is half the battle won, isn't it?

Your 'Why' is Your Compass: A Gentle Nudge Towards Finding Your True North

The age-old quest to understand 'why' - a question that has troubled philosophers for centuries and intermittently fasting individuals for... well, slightly less time.

Determining Your 'Why'

This isn't a mere suggestion; it's an essential step. Why have you chosen to embark on this fasting journey? Is it for tangible health benefits? Is it a strategic approach to weight management? Or perhaps a deeper, personal challenge you've set for yourself? This 'why' is not a fleeting thought; it's the foundation of your fasting journey.

The Importance of Clarity

Imagine setting out on a cross-country road trip without a clear destination in mind. Sure, the idea sounds adventurous, but the reality is that you might end up driving in circles, spending unnecessary time, effort, and resources without truly getting anywhere or enjoying the journey.

Similarly, in our endeavors – whether personal, professional, or, in this case, health-related – clarity is the beacon that lights our path. Let's dive into why clarity, especially regarding intermittent fasting, is so pivotal:

1. **Guided Decision Making:** With clarity, every decision you make becomes purpose driven. When you're clear about why you're undertaking intermittent fasting, you can make informed choices about your diet, fasting windows, and cheat days (which I'm not a fan of, but we'll talk more about that later), aligning them all with your end goal.

2. **Enhanced Focus:** A clear vision ensures you're not easily swayed by distractions or temptations. Remember that slice of cake that calls out to you during your fasting window? Clarity is what helps you smile, decline politely, and move on, keeping your goal in sight.

3. **Emotional Stability:** Let's be real; there will be days that are tougher than others. When hunger strikes or when doubts cloud your mind, clarity is the anchor that reminds you of the bigger picture, allowing you to weather the storm with grace. I personally battle with eating out of boredom and for some reason putting a bite of food in my mouth often follows a situation that makes me angry. I suppose that's using food as a feel-good mechanism and keeping my eye on the prize helps me not do that. In fact, I've put a picture on the refrigerator door to remind me every time I approach the fridge.

4. **Effective Resource Utilization:** When you have clarity about your fasting goals, you can allocate your resources—time, energy, and even money—more efficiently. You'll invest in food, activities, or routines that align with and support your objectives. You may even find yourself breaking the chains of the past with trying new things... which is GREAT!

5. **Empowerment:** Clarity arms you with confidence. When you know exactly why you're on this journey

and what you plan to achieve, you become your own biggest advocate. This self-assurance empowers you to push through challenges and even become an inspiration for others. This, my friends, is the difference between 'hope' and having a plan. Hope is not a plan… a defined path setting yourself up for success in reaching a defined goal is a plan!

6. **Fulfillment and Satisfaction:** Achieving a goal you've clearly defined brings a deeper sense of satisfaction than wandering aimlessly and stumbling upon success. With clarity, every milestone reached, no matter how small, feels like a significant achievement because it aligns perfectly with the path you've charted.

In the grand tapestry of intermittent fasting, clarity isn't just a thread; it's the pattern, the design that gives meaning to the entire piece. By understanding and emphasizing its importance, you're setting yourself up not just for success but for a journey that's enriching at every step.

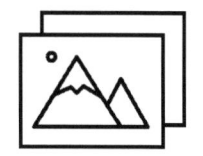

Creating a Vision Board: A Proactive Strategy for Success

A vision board, often brushed off as a crafty endeavor best suited for daydreamers, is in fact a powerful tool in crystallizing and maintaining focus on one's goals. If you're serious about your intermittent fasting journey or any transformative goal for that matter, creating a vision board might be a step worth considering. Here's why:

Visualization: Not Just for Daydreamers!

Now, I've heard some folks say, "Why do I need pictures when I've got imagination?" But trust me on this, there's power in seeing your goals in full Technicolor. It's like the difference between imagining a delicious chocolate cake and having one right in front of you, just begging for a bite. Makes resisting that slice a bit harder, doesn't it? That's the point! Many professional athletes do visioning prior to a game to increase focus and improve outcomes. The player who 'sees' success in their mind realizes it more on the field or court. It's a fact, Jack!

Your Personal Pinterest (Minus the Internet)

Each vision board is a personal story. Your board might have pictures of sprouts and kale because you're on this health spree, or maybe an image of that beach in Bali you're aiming to rock your new, healthy self on. It's a story only you understand - think of it as your personal comic strip, sans the punchlines (unless, of course, you want those in there!).

Making Promises You'll Want to Keep

Setting up a vision board is a bit like promising yourself you'll only eat one cookie and then finding out they're mini-cookies. It's a commitment, but a fun one. Every time you pass by your board, it's a gentle nudge saying, "Remember our deal?" But unlike that cookie pact, this one you'll want to stick to! When you see it, you'll feel it... and keep going!

Evolution, Not Revolution

Your vision board is like a chameleon – ever-changing, adapting. Maybe today it's all about getting those six-pack abs, and a year down the line, it's about mastering the art of mindful eating. The beauty of this is that it is always in flux, just like you. So, if your tastes change from beaches to mountain hikes, no worries – just swap out those photos. No judgment here! Your board SHOULD change. You don't want to be stagnant and keeping your board fresh helps keep you motivated!

For the Feel of it

Let's get sentimental for a second. The act of choosing each image or quote means it resonates with you on some level. It's not just about looking good – it's about feeling good. It's your mini pep rally, your personal cheer squad, all condensed into a board. I started this mission to fit into my skinny jeans. But it didn't take long to realize that seeing the number on the scales drop is just an added benefit to taking on a greater health journey. I found that seeking the best health I can give to myself is a greater reward. It literally moves me to tears if I really dig into what that means for me. I can spend the rest of my life visiting the doctor's office for an hour-long infusion of poison... oh I mean medicine... or I can make healthy choices and overcome that. Now that's a feel-good motivation, big time!

Words that Work

If you're like me and sometimes need a verbal kick to get moving, adding affirmations to your board can be the secret sauce. Not the "I'm a unicorn" kind (unless that's your jam), but powerful, motivating statements that push you forward, reminding you why that last cookie might not be a good idea after all. Sometimes I add a single word. Get curious and look within to see what drives you. Joy. Confidence. Mojo. Swagger. You get it... go ahead, Word Up!

In a nutshell, your vision board is like your personal GPS, but instead of annoyingly saying "recalculating" every time you make a wrong turn, it gently guides you back to your path. A combination of dreams, humor, and a dash of reality – all of which reminds you why you started this journey in the first place.

Expectations VS Reality

Jumping into fasting can often feel like the first day of school. We arrive with crisp notebooks, shiny new pens, and big dreams of acing the year. But, just as school days can be filled with unexpected pop quizzes, the journey of intermittent fasting has its own set of surprises. Let's navigate through the myths and realities of this adventure.

The Myth: "This will be a breeze!"

Why do we even think this? Well, at a glance, intermittent fasting seems deceptively simple. The principle is straightforward: eat during certain hours and don't eat during others. Add to that the plethora of success stories and glowing testimonials online, and it's easy to think, "Hey, they did it without breaking a sweat, so surely I will just coast through!"

"This will be a breeze!" is often rooted in the oversimplification of the process. We see the superficial layer of the practice - just skipping meals - and think, "I skip meals when I'm busy or forgetful. How hard can it be when it's intentional?" But like an iceberg, there's much more beneath the surface of intermittent fasting than meets the eye.

Another contributing factor to this myth is the comparison game. Watching friends or influencers flaunt their success, we might assume that if they can do it effortlessly, so can we. However, every individual's journey is distinct. What appears a breeze for one might be a tempest for another. Additionally, nobody posts about the crappy days, the struggles, the days when the scale went the wrong direction… so often you are seeing only the shiniest of moments and not the truth of it. Don't compare your every-day to their highlight reel!

The reality: The unpredictable ebb and flow of hunger

Hunger, and the accompanying sensation of it, is a multi-faceted phenomenon deeply rooted in human biology. Let's delve deeper into the unpredictable ebb and flow of hunger through a scientific lens:

Neurohormonal Mechanisms

Hunger is intricately regulated by a series of hormones. Two primary ones are ghrelin and leptin. Ghrelin, often termed the "hunger hormone," is produced in the stomach and signals the brain, specifically the hypothalamus, to induce the sensation of hunger. On the contrary, leptin, produced by fat cells, signals satiety. The balance between these hormones, and their subsequent signaling, can fluctuate based on numerous factors, leading to varying intensities and timings of hunger.

We also should realize many things play into our body's internal conversation. When it comes to ghrelin and leptin, our sleep can play a huge role. If we don't get adequate sleep at night, the next day our signals literally get crossed. Ghrelin increases and leptin decreases making us feel more hungry... to the tune of eating between 20-25% more the following day!! This is science, people! It's real... and it's NOT YOUR FAULT. Don't turn on yourself. Rather, make adjustments to have a better day tomorrow. Turn off your screens 30 minutes before bed. Take a melatonin supplement to help you out. Set a bedtime routine you can stick to more often than not. Work toward good sleep habits as another piece to improving your health.

Glucose Levels

Blood glucose levels significantly influence hunger. When blood glucose drops, the body perceives this as a need for fuel, prompting hunger signals. Insulin, a hormone produced in the pancreas, regulates glucose uptake from the blood, but irregularities in insulin response or sensitivity can lead to oscillations in hunger levels. This improves with experience fasting and metabolically switching.

Circadian Rhythms

Our body's internal clock, or circadian rhythm, also plays a role in hunger regulation. For example, the body naturally releases more ghrelin at certain times of the day, like just before meals, which aligns with our typical eating patterns. This will change with your changing eating patterns, but it does take a minute to catch up to you so be prepared on the first few days.

Gut-Brain Axis

The gut and brain communicate constantly, using a complex network of neural connections and signaling molecules. Specific peptides, like peptide YY (PYY) and cholecystokinin (CCK), released post meals from the gut, act on the brain to induce feelings of fullness. Your brain and your gut communicate A LOT more than people realize. Many hormones come from the gut signaling all kinds of things, including hunger or a drive to eat even if it's not perceived as hunger.

External and Environmental Influences

While internal regulatory systems play a significant role, external factors also modulate hunger. Ambient temperature, physical activity, and even visual or olfactory stimuli (like seeing or smelling food) can trigger hunger or alter its intensity. This is a big one for me! I'm the one who will grab a handful of nuts on the way past the jar simply because they're sitting there. I'm not hungry, I just do it without thinking. Bad Bad! I often have to stop myself and have a little self-talk. "You are not even hungry, and this is a mindless habit… now put it down and get your butt busy doing something productive. Chop CHOP!"

Cognitive and Psychological Aspects

Higher cognitive functions, memory, and emotions can also influence hunger. Previous experiences with food, both positive and negative, can modulate hunger responses. Additionally, emotional states, such as stress, can either suppress or enhance hunger, often mediated by hormones like cortisol.

Stress is a big one – you all ever get stressed? Kidding!!! Good gravy, who doesn't stress on occasion!?! This is also something I have had to work at controlling. Finding practices to keep me on the level have made a world of difference. Like sleep, your stress levels can totally derail your efforts when it comes to weight loss. Stress increases cortisol and cortisol stores in the body as belly fat if we don't 'spend it' somehow. If I get stressed, I have to physically move to work through it. Walk and breathe. It's simple but effective.

Adaptation to Dietary Patterns

When one adopts a new eating pattern, such as intermittent fasting, there's an initial phase where the body recalibrates its hunger signaling. As the body adjusts to these new energy intake patterns, there's often a period of heightened hunger sensations, which eventually stabilizes as the body adapts.

In summary, the sensation of hunger is a result of a highly sophisticated and interconnected system of hormones, neural signals, and external influences. Recognizing and understanding the multifactorial nature of hunger, especially during practices like intermittent fasting, can offer a more informed and nuanced approach to managing it.

Tips for Hunger Management

Hunger management during intermittent, or any fasting necessitates a blend of understanding physiological signals, informed dietary choices, and strategic planning. Here are a few practical tips to navigate periods of hunger:

1. **Stay Hydrated:** Drinking adequate water throughout the day is essential. Often, the body can confuse signals of thirst with hunger. Consuming herbal teas can also offer a feeling of satiety. Often adding a pinch of salt and a squeeze of lemon into my water makes a world of difference. The LMNT mineral packs I mentioned previously come into play here as well. These simple adds can be a game changer. It's amazing how great an impact a touch of flavor can have. Black coffee is also allowed during the fasting window since it is effectively a zero calorie beverage.

2. **Prioritize Protein and Fat:** During eating windows, it's crucial to consume foods rich in protein and healthy fats. These nutrients offer sustained energy and have the property of inducing satiety. Don't choose the leanest cut of meat… eat the fat!! Fat is good for your transition into ketosis and fat-burning mode! We've been brainwashed and we must overcome the propaganda that is in our heads.

Mental & Emotional Preparation

Based upon when you came to be on this planet, you likely have messages implanted in your psyche that are not accurate. I grew up hearing fat demonized. Every conceivable item labeled as low fat and reduced fat, every message pushing lean meat as the best choice, things telling us that full-fat products and real butter are bad for us. NO!! They are not bad for us!! They are REAL FOOD! Margarine and pretend butter spreads were created as a cheap way to fatten livestock with inexpensive ingredients... but the animals wouldn't eat it... so they marketed it to us dumb humans and we snagged it right up to save a dollar. Bad Bad! This infuriates me....OK, I'll get off the soapbox.

Protein maintains muscle and fat creates satiety. We also NEED fat to absorb certain fat-soluble vitamins and nutrients. When you are eating Keto or Carnivore, you get exactly these things. If you are not going low carb, you still want to prioritize protein and healthy fat while also adding in nutrient dense veg and complex carbs.

3. **Engage in Activities:** When hunger pangs become pronounced, engaging in an activity or hobby can help shift focus. Activities like reading, walking, or meditation can serve as useful distractions. For me, the activity needs to be active. Taking a walk, playing with the dogs, embarking on some random project with my hubs, simply going outside and experiencing nature... all good stuff.

4. **Practice Mindful Eating:** It is essential to be fully present during meals. By savoring each bite and chewing food thoroughly, one not only enjoys the meal more but also allows the body time to recognize satiety signals. This also prevents overeating simply because you're not paying attention to what or how much you are consuming until you're stuffed to the point of misery.

    Get inside yourself when you eat. I know that sounds strange… but really. What do you smell? What temperature is the food or drink? What texture do you experience on your palette? Take note of the various taste centers on your tongue… sweet, salty, spicy, sour, umami… what do you taste first? Truly experience what you consume. It makes a difference much more than you might imagine. This can create some pretty interesting dinner table conversations too!!!

5. **Avoid Empty Calories:** Consuming sugary or overly processed foods can lead to rapid fluctuations in blood sugar levels, potentially increasing feelings of hunger. It's advisable to consume nutrient-dense foods that offer sustained energy.

    I strongly recommend you cut out sugar as much as you possibly can. Use plant-based sweeteners if you need a sweetener for your coffee, tea, or after-dinner indulgence. I personally tend toward the monk fruit and stevia-based products. The ingredients on the container should all be recognizable. Don't eat sugar substitutes made out of chemicals!!

Cutting out refined wheat/flour has also made a huge impact for me. This reduced the quantity of processed foods I was consuming but also reduced gluten and carbohydrates. For me, this single elimination had the biggest impact on my hunger levels. Once the wheat was gone, I was in control, not the growls in my stomach.

Why? Sugar and carbs spike your blood sugar causing a crash later. When your blood sugar crashes, your body starts screaming at you for more. It's also like a drug in that it gives you a little dopamine hit, the feel-good hormone your body puts out when something is pleasurable. This is why people get addicted to sweets… it really is a literal addiction. I'm not saying it's easy to just put these things down and - poof - it's all better. No. It takes effort. Clean out the fridge and cabinets. Bring in healthy replacements. Don't turn on yourself if you make a mistake … but if you DO take a bite of the doughnut and it's not nearly as delicious as your mind tricked you into believing, don't finish it! Eat blueberries or fresh pineapple instead if you need some sweetness.

6. **Manage Stress:** Elevated stress levels can induce hunger and cravings. Employing techniques like yoga, deep breathing exercises, or journaling can assist in stress reduction. Stress management keeps your cortisol levels down which is tremendously

beneficial to weight management. When your body feels stress, cortisol is produced, and your body reads that as "I'm not safe." Your caveman (caveperson) brain kicks in and triggers the desire to eat so the body can be protected by extra fat stores. You are trying to do just the opposite of this! So, keeping stress to a minimum is huge... work on it!

7. **Ensure Adequate Sleep:** Sleep plays a pivotal role in regulating hormones related to hunger, such as ghrelin and leptin. Obtaining 7-9 hours of sleep is recommended for optimal physiological balance. This one is also tough for many of us. Managing our busy lives comes before our own health too often. I have had to try to improve my 'sleep hygiene' by removing the TV, bright lights, and electronics from the bedroom. I try to maintain a set schedule for bedtime, and I do breathwork as a means to relax and focus my mind to fall asleep. This prevents looping thoughts very well!

8. **Listen to Your Body:** While experiencing hunger is a natural occurrence, if these sensations become overwhelming or lead to discomfort, it may be necessary to adjust the fasting window or seek guidance from a nutrition specialist. Try eating half of an avocado with a bit of salt sprinkled on it and wait 30 minutes. Perhaps your body just needs a little help adjusting. Fat can calm the hunger pangs amazingly well without increasing your insulin which keeps you in your fasted state and allows the benefits to continue and build.

9. **Plan Ahead:** Anticipating fasting periods and scheduling activities or tasks, especially during times one might typically feel hunger, can be beneficial. How does the saying go? 'Fail to plan, plan to fail'... or something like that. In the beginning, this was true for me. I had to set myself up for success by making a plan I could stick to. Like: Today I'm going to fast with my eating window from 4:00 to 8:00 PM and while I'm fasting I'm going to work on XYZ projects for work, take a walk on my mid-day break (notice I didn't say lunch!), and I'll spend 15 minutes doing mindfulness meditation somewhere in my day. If I went into my day with no plan, it was much harder to make good choices. I also took a lemon and a small packet of sea salt to add to my water to ensure I didn't fall off the hydration wagon during the day. All these small things matter!

10. **Stay Connected:** Engaging with others who practice intermittent fasting and exchanging experiences can offer valuable insights and support. Do this with your life partner or a good friend or family member and you've always got someone to talk through things with.

Successful hunger management during fasting hinges on a combination of physiological understanding, informed food choices, and strategic actions. Adhering to these tips can help individuals traverse the fasting periods with greater ease and confidence.

The Grand Vision: Keeping Your Eyes on the Prize

In every endeavor, especially one as personally transformative as embarking on a fasting lifestyle, setting a clear vision can be the very anchor that holds you steadfast amidst the ebbing tides of doubt and uncertainty.

Visualizing End Goals

Science has repeatedly shown that the act of visualization significantly bolsters the chances of success. When we visualize our desired outcome – be it a healthier physique, enhanced mental clarity, or a certain sense of accomplishment – we essentially create a roadmap in our mind. This mental image acts as a compass, continually pointing us toward our north star, ensuring we stay on course. It primes the brain, subconsciously reinforcing the belief that the visualized outcome is attainable, thus propelling us to act in ways that align with our goals.

Celebrating Milestones

The journey of intermittent fasting is not a straight path; it's a series of steps, each deserving of acknowledgment. Recognizing and celebrating milestones, irrespective of their magnitude, serves multiple purposes. Firstly, it provides tangible evidence of progress, which can be a motivating force. Secondly, by celebrating small victories, we cultivate a sense of gratitude and positivity, both of which can be potent fuels for the continued journey. Whether it's sticking to the fasting window for a week straight, resisting a late-night snack, or noticing improved energy levels, each milestone is a testament to progress.

Rewarding Transformation

When one embarks on the journey of intermittent fasting, the immediate vision often revolves around physical transformation. However, as the days turn into weeks and weeks into months, a deeper, more profound change emerges. Beyond the physical, there lies a realm of mental and emotional metamorphosis. Clarity replaces the cloud of mental fog; discipline begins to overshadow momentary impulses; resilience takes the front seat, pushing back fleeting moments of weakness. This all-encompassing transformation becomes one of the most rewarding aspects of the journey. It's a testament to the holistic betterment, a beacon that illuminates not just the external, but the very core of our being.

In essence, the journey of intermittent fasting, bolstered by clear visualization, acknowledgment of progress, and recognition of holistic transformation, becomes more than just a dietary regimen. It evolves into a profound journey of self-discovery, discipline, and growth. Keeping the grand vision in sight ensures that, despite the challenges and fluctuations, one remains unwaveringly committed to the end goal.

Chapter Summary

Hunger is a complex phenomenon governed by a mix of hormones, glucose levels, our body's internal clock, the connection between our gut and brain, environmental factors, psychological aspects, and our eating patterns. Two key hormones, ghrelin and leptin, play major roles in hunger and satiety signaling. Our body's hunger responses can be influenced by a myriad of internal and external factors, making it an unpredictable sensation. When undertaking practices like intermittent fasting, understanding these intricacies can help in managing hunger more effectively.

Successfully navigating hunger during fasting involves both physiological understanding and practical strategies. Key tips include staying hydrated, consuming foods rich in protein and healthy fat, being active, eating mindfully, avoiding foods that cause blood sugar spikes, managing stress, getting adequate sleep, and planning ahead. Connecting with a community and listening to your body's signals can also aid in the journey.

Setting a clear vision is crucial for success in intermittent fasting. Visualization techniques can help in staying focused on end goals. Celebrating small and big milestones is essential for motivation and recognizing progress. While physical transformation is often the immediate goal, the mental and emotional evolution that emerges over time is equally rewarding. This holistic transformation, combined with a clear vision and acknowledgment of progress, makes intermittent fasting a journey of self-discovery and growth.

In a nutshell, the chapter delves into the intricacies of hunger, provides actionable tips to manage it during fasting, and emphasizes the importance of having a clear vision to navigate the challenges and celebrate the transformative rewards of the intermittent fasting journey.

References

1. Clayton, D. J., Mode, W. J. A., & Slater, T. (2020). Optimizing intermittent fasting: Evaluating the behavioral and metabolic effects of extended morning and evening fasting. *Nutrition Bulletin, 45*(4), 444-455.

2. Collier, R. (2013). Intermittent fasting: the science of going without. *Canadian Medical Association Journal, 185*(9), E363-E364.

3. Varady, K. A., Cienfuegos, S., Ezpeleta, M., & Gabel, K. (2022). Clinical application of intermittent fasting for weight loss: progress and future directions. *Nature Reviews Endocrinology, 18*(5), 309-321.

Chapter 4

Fasting Made Easier

Embarking on a fasting journey can seem daunting. However, with some well-considered strategies, it can be a smoother and more manageable process. Let's discuss some effective approaches to make fasting not only easier but also more beneficial.

I've found a few 'hacks' that were true game-changers for me... dare I share? Yes, of course I will! You can sift through these and decide what resonates with you and leave out the rest. Remember, this is not a one-size-fits-all program. This is YOUR strategy that YOU tailor to YOUR LIFE!

Hunger Hacks: Worth A Try

MCT Oil

The magic elixir... MCT Oil is derived from coconuts so it's a healthy fat ... and you can find it everywhere, even Walmart! I recommend you stick to organic varieties that are produced in GMP (good management practices) food manufacturing facilities, but this stuff is quite readily available.

MCT stands for medium chain triglycerides. That's medical lingo for fat! MCT can be converted to Ketones by the liver and cross the blood-brain barrier for fuel. This is a huge asset since the brain cannot store fuel, it requires a steady feed.

I add MCT oil to my morning coffee. You can also simply consume it with a spoon or take the non-glamorous 'swig' from the bottle if you're not sharing it! Ha! Consuming even a tablespoon or two of MCT Oil in the morning provides your system with fuel to last for hours. This will ward off the thoughts of food for quite a while! This one simple trick proved to be the catalyst needed to get several people I worked with moving in the right direction… the needed nudge.

Exogenous Ketones: Fasting Fuel

Ketones are naturally produced by the body when you transition into a fat-burning state. But did you know you can add ketones to the mix from outside sources to boost the fat burn and fuel your brain? It's true! You can find exogenous ketones in liquid or powder forms, choose what you feel is most convenient and/or suited to your needs. I've tried both and they work equally well.

A dose of ketones is like fasting fuel. It provides fuel for your brain, and you feel sharp and able to maintain laser-sharp focus on your task, even if you have not eaten in many hours, days even! It also fuels your body and can provide a boost in performance when you are doing things a bit more physical. My favorite benefit of exogenous ketones… ketones stave off hunger. If I'm feeling that suggestion of hunger but I know I have several more hours before my eating window, a small swig of ketones is all that's needed to hold me over. One shot and the thought of food totally vanishes. Exogenous ketones can also help stabilize blood sugar. They can be taken before bed, and they'll keep your blood sugar pretty flat and not make you feel wound up or jittery at all. The crazy part is you can also take a shot (liquid shot, not an injection) before a workout and you'll feel totally pumped and ready to rock, but again not jacked or jittery like energy drinks or high levels of caffeine might.

I have also seen exogenous ketones help with things that really don't have anything to do with dieting or weight loss. For example, those with anxiety or depression might find ketones beneficial. They help our brains in amazing ways. I've seen people feel more calm than they've felt in years after a drink of ketones, far beyond what any big pharma medicine can do. I've also known women in the throws of perimenopause struggling to sleep due to hormone changes take ketones before bed and get the best sleep they've had in a very long time. Honestly, I can't think of anything ketones don't help!! They're AMAZING. Just beware of fakes and don't break the bank on this stuff… your body makes them for free, remember!

Staying Hydrated: The Role of Water and Herbal Teas

Hydration, especially during fasting, is not merely about quenching thirst but maintaining essential bodily functions. Water is central to nearly every physiological process in our bodies. Here's a deeper dive into the role of water and herbal teas during fasting:

Detoxification

Our bodies are constantly working to remove waste products and toxins. Kidneys, pivotal in this detoxification process, require an ample amount of water to filter out waste from our bloodstream. During fasting, as the intake of other substances is reduced, the body might increase its detoxification processes. This is where water becomes crucial, assisting in flushing out the accumulated toxins through urine.

Metabolism Support

Water plays an indirect yet essential role in metabolism. Various metabolic reactions in our cells require a watery environment. Additionally, water can enhance energy expenditure. A study from the Journal of Clinical Endocrinology and Metabolism found that drinking 500ml of water increased metabolic rate by 30% in both men and women. This suggests that, during fasting, staying hydrated might optimize the metabolic benefits one hopes to achieve.

Hunger Alleviation

Interestingly, the brain sometimes struggles to differentiate between hunger and thirst signals. Dehydration can often manifest as feelings of hunger. By staying hydrated, one might circumvent these false hunger cues, making the fasting period feel less arduous.

Herbal Teas as a Companion

While water is essential, the monotony of it can sometimes be unappealing, especially during extended fasting windows. Herbal teas emerge as an excellent alternative. Not only do they hydrate, but they also bring with them a palette of health benefits.

For instance, chamomile tea is renowned for its calming effects. It's been traditionally used to alleviate anxiety and induce sleep. During fasting, when mood fluctuations might be more pronounced, a cup of chamomile can be grounding.

Peppermint tea, on the other hand, is a boon for the digestive system. It's known to reduce bloating and soothe digestive discomfort. As the digestive system gets a break during fasting, peppermint tea can further optimize this rest period, ensuring smoother digestion once the fast is broken.

While fasting is an abstention from food, it emphasizes the importance of hydration. Whether it's plain water or a comforting herbal brew, ensuring adequate fluid intake is paramount for a successful and comfortable fasting experience.

Nourishing Foods for Breaking Fast

After a period of fasting, the body is in a unique metabolic state. The regular influx of nutrients has been paused, and the body has likely tapped into its reserves to fuel itself. Therefore, how you reintroduce food becomes pivotal, not just for immediate well-being but also for maximizing the benefits of the fast.

The Role of Proteins

Proteins are the building blocks of our bodies. They're crucial for repairing and building tissues, producing enzymes and hormones, and other essential bodily functions. When you consume protein-rich foods like grass-fed meats after a fast, you're essentially supplying your body with essential amino acids it needs for these processes. Moreover, proteins have a satiating effect. This means you'll feel full and satisfied, reducing the likelihood of overeating post-fast. Do buy the highest quality meat you can. Grass fed, grass finished beef is top quality. But if that's out of your price range, choose the best you can afford.

Importance of Healthy Fats

Fats, often misunderstood, are vital for our health. They're essential for absorbing certain vitamins (like A, D, E, and K) and producing hormones. Healthy fats, like those found in avocados, coconuts, or olive oil, also provide a sustained energy source. Unlike the quick and fleeting energy spikes associated with sugars, fats offer a more stable and lasting energy release.

The #1 thing you can do to improve cellular function is eliminate bad fats!! Healthy fats are a subject I could really go on and on about… but I'll try to keep it direct and to the point here. Fats derived from the fruit of the plant are healthy fats. These include olive oil, avocado oil, and coconut oil. Fats from the seeds of the plant, corn oil, soybean oil, and so on are bad fats. The 'badness' is in the amount of linoleic acid, an omega 6 fatty acid, they contain. The seed oils are by far the highest in linoleic acid, sometimes by 10-fold or more when compared to the healthier oil selections.

Linoleic acid mucks up the bilipid layer (double layer of fat) that surrounds our cells. The mitochondria and working parts inside the cell need to be able to transfer nutrients in, waste out, and stay protected inside their cellular membrane, the bilipid layer. When seed oils high in linoleic acid are taken into the body the pathways that allow for the transfers in and out of the cells get gummed up, plugged with muck if you will. Sometimes it can take years for the body to eliminate this sludge. This is best avoided so much as possible. How do you avoid the bad oils? Choose avocado oil, coconut oil, or olive oil to use in your home. And don't eat fried foods in restaurants.

Complex Carbohydrates are Better

Carbohydrates are the body's primary energy source. However, not all carbohydrates are created equal. Simple carbs, like those in candies or sodas, give a rapid spike in blood sugar, followed by a steep crash, leading to fluctuating energy levels. On the contrary, complex carbohydrates, found in foods like whole grains and sweet potatoes, break down slowly. This results in a steady release of glucose into the bloodstream, ensuring consistent energy levels. Moreover, complex carbs are typically high in fiber, promoting gut health and further aiding in satiety.

Blood Sugar Stability

The foods you eat after fasting can have a direct impact on your blood sugar levels. Spiking blood sugar levels can lead to energy surges followed by lethargy, and over time, can stress the body's insulin response mechanism. By choosing proteins, healthy fats, and complex carbs, you're ensuring a more balanced and gradual rise in blood sugar. This not only feels better but is also healthier for the body.

In summary, breaking a fast is more than just eating the first thing you see. It's about nourishing the body with what it genuinely needs. By opting for a balanced combination of proteins, healthy fats, and complex carbohydrates, you're laying down the foundation for optimal post-fast recovery and sustained well-being.

Exercise and Movement During Fasting

The concept of fasting often conjures up images of stillness and inactivity, given the reduced caloric intake. However, integrating gentle movement into this phase can offer multifold benefits.

Circulatory Boost

Movement, even if subtle, stimulates the circulatory system. Blood, the lifeline of our body, carries oxygen and vital nutrients to cells and removes waste products. By engaging in activities like walking or stretching, you're facilitating this process, ensuring efficient nutrient delivery and waste elimination. Enhanced circulation also aids in reducing feelings of sluggishness that can sometimes accompany fasting.

Increased Autophagy & Deeper Ketosis

Exercise during fasting can further advance the benefits you are fasting to achieve. Listen to your body while adding in exercise so as not to push too far too fast. Take things gentle at first and work your way into a more advanced exercise if that's your preference. If you get lightheaded or start having unusual sensations or heart palpitations, definitely stop and assess the situation. Once you are comfortable with exercise during fasting, you can use exercise to more quickly burn through the carbs and sugar in your system and more quickly enter ketosis and initiate autophagy.

Mood Enhancement

Physical movement, especially practices like yoga, or even dancing, have profound effects on the endocrine system. Engaging in these activities stimulates the release of endorphins, which are naturally occurring chemicals in the body that promote feelings of well-being and happiness. They're often dubbed the body's "natural painkillers" and can elevate mood. For someone who's fasting, this is particularly beneficial as it counteracts potential mood dips or feelings of irritability due to hunger.

Mitigation of Hunger Pangs

Engaging in gentle activities offers a productive distraction from the sensation of hunger. The focus shifts from the void in the stomach to the movement of the body. Furthermore, there's a biological angle to this. Exercise stimulates the release of peptide YY (PYY), a hormone produced in the gut in response to eating, which has been shown to increase feelings of fullness. So, paradoxically, some forms of movement might alleviate hunger during fasting.

Cognitive Benefits

The benefits of movement aren't just physical. Gentle exercises, especially those that require mindfulness like yoga, can sharpen focus and improve cognitive function. This is attributed to the increased blood flow to the brain and the meditative aspects of such practices. During fasting, when one might experience moments of mental fog, these activities can act as a clarifying force.

Diversion from Food Thoughts

Let's face it, during fasting, it's not uncommon for the mind to drift towards thoughts of food. Engaging in activities can serve as a valuable diversion. Instead of obsessively pondering over the next meal, one finds solace and engagement in the rhythm of movement.

While fasting inherently implies a reduction or abstention from food, it doesn't necessarily imply a complete halt in physical activity. Incorporating gentle movements can make the fasting journey more holistic, ensuring that the mind and body stay active and nourished, even in the absence of food.

Adapting Fasting to Energy Levels

Fasting, at its core, is not a one-size-fits-all endeavor, have I mentioned that yet?. Just as our energy levels fluctuate from day to day based on a myriad of factors - from sleep quality to stress levels - the approach to fasting should be equally dynamic.

Body's Feedback Loop

One of the marvels of the human body is its innate feedback mechanism. It constantly communicates its state and needs, often through subtle signs. A sudden drop in energy, mood swings, or even sharper hunger pangs can all be indicators that the body is seeking some adjustments. Paying attention to these cues is paramount, especially when adopting a practice as transformative as fasting.

Importance of Nutrient-Dense Meals

When we talk about adjusting fasting based on energy levels, the focus isn't just on the duration of the fasting window but also on the quality of meals when you break the fast. On days when you sense your energy is on the lower end, it becomes crucial to consume foods that are packed with nutrients. Opt for meals that offer a balanced blend of macronutrients - proteins, healthy fats, and complex carbohydrates. Additionally, ensure you're incorporating micronutrient-rich foods that supply essential vitamins and minerals. This helps in replenishing the body more efficiently.

Flexibility Over Rigidity

There's a misconception that fasting is about strict adherence to set windows of eating and not eating. While consistency can be beneficial, it's equally important to remember that rigidity can lead to burnout. If one day, you feel the need to adjust your fasting hours, it doesn't mean you've strayed from your goals. In fact, being adaptable can enhance your fasting experience, making it more sustainable in the long run.

I would recommend getting comfortable with being flexible, even. Perhaps a group at work invites you to lunch... don't blow them off, go... honestly, GO and enjoy it! Have something light... a nice garden salad or a fruit plate. Then just make an adjustment to your eating window to compensate. There is no such thing as a failed fast. If you pivot, that's OK.

I can't stress this enough... learn to flex, to pivot. Try different fasts. Start with intermittent fasting and slowly push your first meal of the day back an hour, then two. Soon you'll be doing 16/8 like a champ. Next you can try a 24 hour fast. Just keep trying new things. Don't get hung up on only one method. You'll thank yourself later!

The Psychological Aspect

Beyond the physical realm, adapting fasting to energy levels has psychological implications. By allowing oneself the flexibility to adjust, you cultivate a sense of self-compassion. Instead of berating yourself for not sticking to a rigid window, you acknowledge your body's needs and respond with care. This nurtures a healthier relationship with fasting and with oneself.

In conclusion, fasting is as much a journey of self-awareness as it is a dietary practice. By tuning in to one's energy levels and being willing to adapt, you create a fasting regimen that's not only effective but also respectful of your body's ever-changing needs. It underscores the principle that fasting is not a punitive act, but a practice in tune with the body's rhythms.

When to Pause or Modify Fasting Practice

Embarking on the journey of intermittent fasting can sometimes feel like charting a course through unexplored territory, with new experiences and discoveries at each turn. While the pathway towards rejuvenated health and well-being is exciting, it's important to remember that this expedition comes with a 'stop and assess' clause, a moment to recalibrate and perhaps choose a different fork in the road if necessary.

Firstly, let's talk about the vital self-check system that should be in place during fasting. Just like a vigilant ship's captain constantly monitors various parameters to ensure smooth sailing, individuals practicing fasting should be observant of the varied signals their body and mind are emitting. This vigilance forms the cornerstone of a successful and healthy fasting regimen.

One clear signal to possibly reconsider your current fasting strategy is persistent fatigue. This isn't the usual tiredness that everyone feels now and then, but a kind of lethargy that clings to you, reducing your usual zest and energy. This might indicate that your body is asking for a more gradual approach to fasting or a modification in your fasting schedule.

Another signpost indicating that it might be time to pause or adjust is irritability. Now, we are not talking about the minor annoyance one feels when the coffee isn't quite right, but a persistent undercurrent of irritability that seems to color your days. This could potentially be a signal from your brain, indicating that it's feeling the strain and perhaps needs a more nourishing environment to function optimally.

A red flag that is hard to ignore is difficulty concentrating. If you find your attention span dwindling and tasks that usually don't require much effort suddenly seem like scaling mountains, it's time to step back and reassess. Your cognitive function should ideally flourish with a well-planned fasting regimen, and any persistent downturn in this area warrants a second look at your fasting blueprint.

Now, talking about the physical signs, if your digestive system starts sending out SOS signals in the form of severe digestive issues, it's imperative to heed them. Digestive discomfort, persistent issues, or abnormalities are clear indicators that your current fasting regimen might not be in sync with your digestive system's rhythm and capabilities.

Fasting is indeed a promising pathway to enhanced health and vitality, but it should never be at the cost of your well-being. Recognizing the signs that suggest a need for change and responding with agility and wisdom is not a detour in your journey, but an essential part of steering towards a destination of holistic health and well-being. Remember, the fasting journey is not a sprint but a marathon, where pacing, pausing, and sometimes changing tracks, can lead to a more enriching and successful journey.

Fasting and Your Lifestyle

Fasting might initially appear to be a monastic practice, reserved for those with the luxury to mold their day around their dietary patterns. In reality, fasting, with its myriad benefits, can seamlessly weave into the vibrant tapestry of our modern lives, complementing our varying routines, commitments, and adventures. Here's a glimpse into how fasting can harmonize with different facets of contemporary life:

When you think of fasting and travel, your initial reaction might be that they're at odds with each other. After all, traveling, whether for work or pleasure, often comes with a set of unpredictable elements - flight delays, jet lag, or even unexpected local delicacies. But what if I told you that fasting, especially intermittent fasting, could be your trusty travel companion?

Adaptable Nature of Intermittent Fasting

Intermittent fasting's core strength is its flexibility. It isn't a diet that restricts what you eat but rather when you eat. For the traveler, this means you can adjust your fasting window to accommodate different time zones or travel schedules. Got a long-haul flight from New York to Tokyo? That's essentially a ready-made fasting window. You can initiate your fast a few hours before your flight and break it once you've landed and settled, turning potential flight-induced meal disruptions into a planned fasting period.

Busy Days and Aligning Your Eating Window

Travel often comes with its share of chaos and unexpected turns. If you foresee a day jam-packed with meetings, sightseeing, or just general running around, align your eating window to a time when you can actually sit down and savor your meal. This not only ensures that you maintain your fasting routine but also guarantees a mindful, relaxed eating experience – even if it's just a quick half-hour. Starting your fast earlier the previous evening can be a game-changer on such days, ensuring you get quality nutrition before the whirlwind starts.

Freedom from Constant Meal Planning

One of the most liberating aspects of fasting, especially when on the move, is the absence of the constant need to plan out meals. When you're navigating through unfamiliar places or tight schedules, the last thing you want is the added pressure of fitting in three meals. Fasting offers the mental peace of not always scouting for the next meal, allowing you more time to immerse yourself in the moment, be it a crucial business meeting or a mesmerizing sunset.

To sum it up, while the notion of combining fasting and travel might seem counterintuitive at first, it can be an incredibly synergistic duo with the right approach. Intermittent fasting's adaptable nature allows travelers and busy individuals to find a rhythm that works for them, ensuring they get the best of both worlds - the benefits of fasting and the joy of travel or accomplishing tasks on a hectic day.

Social Events and Fasting

Socializing often centers around food and drinks, a universal way humans have connected for ages. So, when you're fasting, it might seem like you're facing an uphill battle. The lavish spreads, the clinking glasses, the tempting aromas - how do you reconcile this with your fasting schedule? Thankfully, with some foresight and strategy, you can enjoy the best of both worlds.

Strategizing for Social Events

Anticipation is key. If you're privy to a social gathering in advance, you can adjust your eating window to coincide with the event. For instance, if there's a dinner party at 7 PM, you could set your eating window from 3 PM to 11 PM, allowing you ample time to enjoy the festivities. This approach means you're not just sitting there, poking at your food-less plate while others dive into their meals. Instead, you're in the thick of the action, savoring the meal and the company.

When the Fast Doesn't Break

What if you find yourself at an impromptu gathering or an event that falls squarely in your fasting phase? First, don't panic. Instead, pivot. There's always an array of beverages that can be your companion. Sparkling water with a squeeze of lemon can feel both refreshing and festive. Unsweetened teas, be it green or herbal, offer flavor without breaking your fast. But beyond that, redirect your attention to the heart of the gathering: the people. Engage in conversations, dance if there's music, or simply cherish the joyous ambiance.

Embracing the Non-food Aspects

Food, while central to many gatherings, is just one facet. There's laughter, stories, debates, and countless shared moments that don't revolve around the dining table. Instead of feeling restricted by your fasting window, view it as an opportunity to truly soak in these moments. With food out of the equation, even temporarily, you might find yourself listening more intently, laughing a little harder, and connecting on a deeper level.

While fasting can seem at odds with our inherently social nature, it doesn't have to be. With a mix of planning and a shift in perspective, you can successfully interweave your social endeavors with your fasting commitments, ensuring neither takes a backseat. The result? A richer, more fulfilling social experience, both gastronomically and emotionally.

Fasting and Nutrition

While the spotlight often shines on the 'not eating' aspect of fasting, the periods when you do eat are just as crucial, if not more so. In fact, this is where the magic happens. The way you nourish your body during your eating windows can make all the difference in how you experience and benefit from fasting. It's like owning a luxury car - you wouldn't dream of filling it with low-quality fuel, would you? Similarly, your body, during fasting, is in a heightened state, and it's imperative to provide it with premium fuel.

Quality Over Quantity

Given the limited eating window during intermittent fasting, it might be tempting to indulge in calorie-rich foods to 'make up' for the missed meals. However, this mindset can be counterproductive. It's not about cramming in calories, but about choosing nutrient-dense foods. This means embracing foods rich in vitamins, minerals, fiber, proteins, and healthy fats. It's about colorful vegetables, clean proteins, some whole grains, and beneficial fats like those from avocados and nuts. Like removing toxins, seek to eat the best you can afford. You don't need a $30 steak for dinner multiple days each week. But eating clean, grass fed / grass finished beef goes a long way in toxin avoidance.

The Mindset Shift

When you view fasting from a perspective of deprivation, you risk turning it into a grueling task. But when you see it as an opportunity—a chance for your body to rest, repair, and rejuvenate—your approach to nutrition during eating windows evolves. You begin to see meals as opportunities to nourish and heal, rather than just satiate hunger. Your mindset can make you or break you here. This can be said for most things, really. Rather than focusing on what you are NOT having, focus on what you ARE having and the amazing benefits you are experiencing from it. Celebrate your awesomeness and how you are practicing self-love through nourishing your body well. Say it with me… I LOVE MY BODY!!

Signaling Care to Your Body

Our bodies are incredible machines, capable of phenomenal feats. But like any machine, they need proper maintenance. By ensuring you get quality nutrition during your eating windows, you're sending a powerful message to your body: "I value you. I care for you."

This positive reinforcement not only aids in physical health but also bolsters mental and emotional well-being. Repeat after me… I LOVE ME!! I LOVE ME!! I LOVE AND VALUE MY AMAZING BODY!! ☺

Sustainability and Enrichment

For fasting to be a sustainable practice, it shouldn't feel like punishment. It should feel like a routine that's both enriching and rejuvenating. By prioritizing proper nutrition, you ensure that fasting becomes a practice that you look forward to, rather than dread. Over time, this balance between fasting and nutrition cultivates a deeper understanding and respect for one's body, its needs, and its incredible resilience.

In essence, fasting is only half the story. The other half is how you choose to break the fast. A balanced approach, prioritizing quality nutrition, transforms intermittent fasting from a mere dietary regimen to a holistic practice that nourishes the mind, body, and soul.

Chapter Summary

Making fasting Easier delves into the varied strategies that can simplify the intermittent fasting experience. Foremost among these is the importance of staying hydrated. Consuming water throughout the fasting window can significantly mitigate feelings of hunger. Herbal teas, offering a departure from the monotony of plain water, not only provide variety but also play a role in aiding digestion and further suppressing appetite.

As fasting comes to an end, the foods chosen to break it become pivotal. The emphasis here is on nourishing foods, particularly those that are whole and unprocessed. These foods, packed with nutrients, deliver steady energy and prevent rapid fluctuations in blood sugar levels. This is especially important to counteract the potential for overeating or choosing less nutritious options in response to intense hunger.

Exercise and movement, albeit gentle forms, are also championed during fasting periods. Activities like walking, stretching, or yoga can boost circulation, elevate mood, and serve as a distraction from hunger pangs. Moreover, being attuned to the body's signals is integral to a successful fasting experience. Recognizing and differentiating between feelings of hunger and fullness can serve as a roadmap to navigate the fasting journey.

Furthermore, the adaptability of fasting is underscored, emphasizing the importance of adjusting the regimen based on one's energy levels. If fasting feels too draining or if energy levels wane, it may be time to reconsider the fasting window or the nutrient density of meals. Additionally, it's crucial to stay vigilant for any negative signs or symptoms. If adverse effects become evident, be they physical, mental, or emotional, one should be prepared to modify or even pause their fasting routine.

Fasting and Your Lifestyle extends the conversation on fasting into the realm of daily routines and scenarios. Traveling or navigating through busy days needn't disrupt fasting schedules. With some foresight, fasting can be tailored to align with travel times or less hectic parts of the day. Similarly, social events can be managed by adjusting eating windows or employing strategies that allow one to partake in the festivity without necessarily indulging in food.

Integrating fasting into an everyday routine might seem daunting, but with structured planning and an understanding of one's body, it can become second nature. The chapter also places importance on shared experiences. Personal accounts from varied individuals illuminate the journey of fasting, highlighting the shared challenges faced and the lessons imbibed.

Finally, a crucial aspect of fasting is the balance of nutrition. Ensuring the intake of nutrient-rich foods, being aware of micronutrient requirements during fasting, and resisting the urge to overindulge after fasting are all vital components of a balanced fasting practice. The overall essence of the chapter lies in providing comprehensive guidance on making intermittent fasting not just manageable but also a beneficial and integrated part of one's lifestyle.

References

1. Food Addiction and Intermittent Fasting. (2020). *Journal of Addiction Research, 4*(1).

2. The whys and wherefores of intermittent fasting. (2021). *Knowable Magazine.* https://doi.org/10.1146/knowable-052021-2

3. Clayton, D. J., Mode, W. J. A., & Slater, T. (2020). Optimizing intermittent fasting: Evaluating the behavioral and metabolic effects of extended morning and evening fasting. *Nutrition Bulletin, 45*(4), 444-455.

4. Niepoetter, P., Butts-Wilmsmeyer, C., & Gopalan, C. (2022). Intermittent fasting and mental and physical fatigue in obese and non-obese rats. *PLOS ONE, 17*(11), e0275684.

5. Nair, P., & Khawale, P. (2016). Role of therapeutic fasting in women's health: An overview. *Journal of Mid-Life Health, 7*(2), 61.

6. Horne, B. D., Muhlestein, J. B., & Anderson, J. L. (2015). Health effects of intermittent fasting: hormesis or harm? A systematic review. *The American Journal of Clinical Nutrition, 102*(2), 464-470.

7. Maslov, P. Z., Sabharwal, B., Ahmadi, A., Baliga, R., & Narula, J. (2022). Religious fasting and the vascular health. *Indian Heart Journal, 74*(4), 270-274.

Sample Fasting Schedules

Fasting Method	Fasting Window	Eating Window	Sample Schedule
16/8 Method (Lean-gains)	16 hours	8 hours	First meal at 12:00 PM, end at 8:00 PM.
14/10 Method	14 hours	10 hours	First meal at 8:00 AM, end at 6:00 PM.
5:2 Diet	2 days (limited cals)	5 days (normal)	Normal eating for 5 days, 500-600 calories on 2 days.
Eat-Stop-Eat	24 hours	–	Dinner at 7:00 PM, don't eat until 7:00 PM next day.
Alternate-Day Fasting	24 hours (every other day)	Alternate days	Fast from Monday night to Tuesday night, etc.
20/4 Method (Warrior Diet)	20 hours	4 hours	Small fruits/veggies during the day, larger meal 6:00 PM to 10:00 PM.
One Meal A Day (OMAD)	23 hours	1 hour	One large meal, e.g., at 6:00 PM.
Random Meal Skipping	–	–	No fixed pattern, skip meals when convenient.

Getting Started Methods

Once again in case I haven't mentioned it… there is no one size fits all here! Ha! That said, I wanted to put a few sets of optional guidelines here at the end to choose from to help you get started. These are guidelines and not set in stone, of course. And these are totally optional, flexible, and customizable to your needs.

I know when I was just starting out on my health journey, everything was totally trial and error. Which is fine, you learn things that way. But it sure would have been great to make quicker progress toward my goals. That very thing is the aim of this chapter. Let's lay down some bumpers we can aim to stay between to keep us on the path toward success. Ready? Heck to the yah you are! ☺

Becoming Metabolically Flexible

First, let's start with the path I took. I read over and over again how powerful a weight loss strategy it can be to combine intermittent fasting with keto or carnivore style eating. So that's where I stepped in. The more I learned, the more I found that I was actually becoming metabolically flexible at the same time… bonus! Once your body can switch between using carbs or ketones for fuel, all styles of fasting becomes tremendously easier.

What does getting fat adapted or metabolically flexible entail, you ask? It's essentially going as fully into a keto or carnivore type eating plan – I like to call my style of eating Ketovore, somewhere between the two - long enough to allow your body to switch over to using ketones for energy. For some this can happen in a week if your carb count stays low enough. Others I've worked with might take up to two or three weeks. We have to realize we've been eating pizza and fast food for A LONG TIME! To see our bodies flip over to fat-burning mode in less than a month is pretty impressive, if you ask me! We all love instant gratification but remember this is a long game we are playing for overall health. Anything worth doing is worth doing for more than a week!

Step 1: Remove sugar, things made from wheat (bread, pasta, cake, etc.), and veggies high in starch (corn, potatoes, etc.) from your diet.

Step 2: Read the label on EVERYTHING you buy that comes in a package. Seek to keep your daily carb count between 20 and 50 grams. I like to shoot for 25 just to have a solid goal in mind. This can be challenging if you've not eaten this way before!!

Step 3: Focus on whole foods. Shop around the outer aisles of the grocery store. Buy meats, cheese, full-fat dairy, and lots of fresh vegetables. You can also include fresh fruits as long as mind your total carbs. While eating this way, don't buy low fat or fat free… you want the fat. It helps you feel satisfied and gives your fat-burning engines some fuel to get the process started.

Step 4: You'll know your body has flipped over to fat-burning when you feel like you are no longer hungry. Yep, you read that correctly. It's an amazing thing. You'll suddenly realize that you have to remind yourself to eat because your body is taking care of business without asking you for any input at all. You'll be able to go for much longer without food than you might imagine at this point. This is a great time start stretching out your fasting window. Push your first meal of the day back until lunch, or even later if you can. You may even find yourself able to do OMAD - One Meal A Day - for a few days to see how that suits your lifestyle.

And your fasting begins! Once you've reached this point, you can play with fasting options and find what works for you. I highly recommend you don't go too far too fast. And give your body some practice switching between fuel systems. Stay in fat-burn for a week, then have a carb day and eat rice, sweet potatoes, or other complex carbs for a day or two. I typically don't go for 'cheat days' because I feel like we only cheat ourselves when we make bad choices. Carbs are not bad. We want carbs sometimes. So, a day or two with higher carb counts does not include pizza and donuts for me. Those things are health bombs, not cheat meals.

Remember, this is all built around your favorite foods, your schedule, your life! YOU ARE IN CONTROL!

Intermittent Fasting; No Dietary Changes

Some people I have worked with have no intention of changing to a keto or carnivore style of eating. Their food choices tend mostly to carbohydrates, and they don't want to make drastic changes. Ok… that's fine too. Fasting is totally flexible and can work with any eating style you choose!! This style of getting started has less steps and can be initiated by anyone any time as long as you work into it gradually.

Step 1: Choose your fasting goal – do you want to start out with a 14-hour fasting window, 12-hour? Once you determine the length of fast you want, you can choose where that should start and stop. If you are doing a 12-hour fasting window… you might finish your last meal of the day at 8PM and you would not eat anything again until 8AM – that's a 12 hour fast! Pretty simple, right!?! And for this style of Intermittent Fasting, you eat as you always have, you just keep the food intake within your feeding window.

Step 2: If you want to increase the length of your fasts, do it gradually. Start with a 12 or 14 hour fast and stick to that for a few days. Once you're comfortable with that, open it up another hour for a few days… and so on. This style of IF can be turned on and off to suit your day and your schedule as needed. No significant changes are made to your diet.

Sending You Much Love and Grace – Final Words

You are all amazing humans. You live in a miraculous body that has astonishing capabilities this modern world has lost sight of. When you take your health into your own hands, as you are doing, you truly learn about yourself and what you are capable of on a much deeper level.

Focus on your health, not on a number on the scale. In fact, I rarely weigh in. I go by how I feel, how my clothes fit, how much energy and resilience I have. I know we don't live in the land of perfect - far from it for most of us. But if we could have a closer relationship with nature and where our food comes from, that would be a tremendous health boost. Seek out your local farmer's market. Know the name of the nice people you buy farm-fresh eggs and produce from. Your kids should know where the foods they eat come from. In fact, let them grow something and eat it! Even if it's just in a flowerpot on the ledge, it makes the connection to nature.

Don't get hung up on any one thing. Become flexible and fluid. Change things up, as nature intended. Eat with the seasonal offerings. Eat for nourishment over all else. When you have a colorful plate of nutrient dense foods prepared with love, nothing tastes better! Share this with someone and enjoy the boost of

Oxytocin, the feel-good hormone! Change up your activities. Don't get stuck in a rut of rinse & repeat. Your life is ever-changing and the way you approach your food and activity should mirror that. There is no right answer that suits everyone. We all have to find what works for us. So many things go into good health, food is just one of them.

Your mental state plays a huge role in your health too! Take time to de-stress. Have create a self-love and gratitude practice. When you set an intention to find the things you are grateful for each day, your perspective begins to shift in that direction. When the vehicle cuts you off in traffic, perhaps they're having an emergency – you never know. Give them some grace too! Breathe. Do yoga. Walk in nature. Pet your dog or cat. Have a glass of wine with your bestie. Spend a candle-lit evening with someone you love. Sit and talk with your parents or grandparents. Surprise someone with a bouquet of flowers for no particular reason.

Start a journal or a simple bullet list of where you are. You can periodically update things and see your WINS. Take your power back by giving yourself some momentum. Take a holistic approach to your health. Trust yourself. Have confidence in yourself. Be curious… about food, about places to see, about all things! Work to eliminate negative self-talk inside your head. Start finding and saying out loud one thing you love about yourself each day. Say it loud!

Live – Love – Laugh!! And don't forget to love YOURSELF!!

Made in the USA
Columbia, SC
27 July 2024